DAILY
BREAD

DAILY BREAD

What Kids Eat Around the World

Gregg Segal

Foreword by
Bee Wilson

pH powerHouse Books Brooklyn, NY

Introduction
Gregg Segal

Four years ago, I asked family, friends, and neighbors to save their garbage for a week and then lie down and be photographed in it. I figured it would be hard to ignore the problem of consumption and waste when surrounded by your own trash. The most disturbing thing about the garbage was the amount of packaging people went through each week, myself included. While it's true that most of this packaging is recyclable, recycling has a cost and a mighty large carbon footprint.

As I edited *7 Days of Garbage*, I thought about how our diets have been impacted by this revolution in the way food is produced and consumed. There's been a lot of press about skyrocketing obesity rates and handwringing about the causes and what to do. It struck me that one reason we don't give enough thought to what's in our food is because we're not the ones making it! It's that simple. We've outsourced this vital part of our lives, the connective tissue that bonds families and culture. We often choose foods that are ready made, inexpensive, and satiating. But are they nutritious?

I thought, what if we kept a journal of everything we eat and drink for one week to bring our focus onto diet and health in a way that registers and allows us to take ownership of the food we eat. Beginning with kids made sense because eating habits start young. If you don't get it right when you're 9 or 10, it's going to be a lot harder when you're older!

I began shooting in my own backyard, photographing my son Hank and some of his friends from school and then broadened the piece to include kids from other communities in Los Angeles. But the story had only begun. Globalization is altering our relationship to food on every continent. I was driven to find out if and where regional cuisine still thrives and where it's been overrun by burgers, pizza, and chicken nuggets. I launched a Kickstarter, which got me to Mumbai and Kuala Lumpur.

I was surprised to find that in India and Malaysia and other parts of the world, it's not the poor who are the biggest consumers of junk food; in Mumbai, the $13 it costs for a medium Dominoes pizza is beyond the means of most. Local Indian junk food is cheap, but doesn't have cache. Western fast food is appealing for its status as much as its taste.

Fast food has made huge inroads in the Middle East where obesity rates are double world averages. Thirty years ago, diabetes barely existed in this part of the world, but by 2014, there were 803,900 diabetics in the UAE, nearly 20 percent of the population.

In 2015, Cambridge University conducted an exhaustive study ranking diets around the world from most to least nutritional. Remarkably, 9 of the 10 healthiest countries are in Africa. It seems counterintuitive that some of the poorest countries in the world have among the healthiest diets. But when you look closely at what they're eating, it makes sense: fresh vegetables, fruits, nuts, seeds, grains, fish, and legumes and few empty calories (processed, packaged junk foods). Many of the countries with the world's best diets like Chad and Sierra Leone (numbers 1 and 2 on the Cambridge list), are dangerous and have poor infrastructure, so the food giants haven't figured out how to set up their supply chains.

But corporate food is finding ways to profit from even the poorest consumers, reaching remote places that don't have traditional distribution channels. In Brazil, Nestle is hiring "micro-entrepreneurs," mom and pops who peddle cheap, processed foods in remote villages. A generation ago, Brazil's poor were underfed. Now, they have a new problem: 57% of the population is overweight.

One region Nestle won't reach is the Xingu National Park, an indigenous territory of Brazil, its biodiversity protected from encroaching cattle farms and deforestation. The park, in the south of the Amazonian basin, is home to 9-year-old Kawakanih and her tribe, the Yawalapiti, whose traditional way of life is preserved. Kawakanih's daily bread is manioc, a potato-like root that's ground into flour and used to make beiju, a sort of cassava pancake. Kawakanih wraps her beiju around fresh fish caught in the Xingu River. She snacks throughout the day, picking Brazil nuts and wild fruits like pequi and pupunha.

A few hundred miles from Kawakanih, in the Cerrado, a tropical savannah east of the Amazon, Ademilson Francisco dos Santos, 10, harvests fruits and nuts, too. His family farms rice, beans, sesame seeds, pumpkin, manioc, and sweet potato and harvests vanilla trees for medicine. Ademilson's mother makes porridge from baru nuts and jatobá flour. She roasts sesame seeds and grinds them with a mortar and pestle to make Ademilson's favorite treat, paçoca.

There are communities throughout the world where slow food will never be displaced by junk food, where home-cooked meals are the bedrock of family and culture, and where love and pride are sensed in the aromas of stews and curries.

In Catania, Sicily, Amelia Govia is surrounded by vibrant, colorful foods:

green beans, plump cherry tomatoes, radicchio, peppers, zucchini, melon, and peaches. In the Mediterranean, people are willing to spend a larger portion of their income on fresh produce from the farmers market rather than filling their freezers with packaged foods. In fact, outside of a single pizza box, you don't see any packaging in Amelia's meals; everything is homemade, which is not only pleasing to the eye, but easy on the environment. The more we prepare our own meals from whole foods, the less waste and litter we generate.

Seeing a week's worth of food from a bird's-eye perspective allows us to grasp, in one glance, what our diet looks like and what may be missing. In Mumbai, Adveeta Venkatesh's father watched the pictures come up on my laptop as I was shooting. He shook his head and said, "I can't believe Adveeta is eating all that junk! I'm going to have to talk with her mother!" A single mom in Los Angeles took a look at all the junk food in her daughter's diet and confided that her ex-husband was to blame. "Except for that broccoli! That was the night she was home with me!" Parents are blaming each other all over the world because of this project, which tells me that it's helping to move the needle on diet.

The collaboration extends, beyond the picture-taking process, to viewers. I encourage school curriculums to adopt the "Daily Bread Challenge." Students keep track of everything they eat for a week, documenting and breaking down their meals. Which foods are whole and which are processed? How many of the foods they eat have a commercial? How many foods come straight from the garden (or farm) and which come from a package? How many have more than five ingredients? How many of the ingredients can they pronounce? How many colors are represented in their foods? Are there any greens in their diet?

Less than 1% of our calories come from vegetables in the US. Looking at all of the kids' food I photographed, not just in the US, but all over the world, greens were consistently absent. I often hear parents say, with resignation, "My kid won't eat vegetables." They often throw up their hands. "She only likes plain pasta." And bacon. And fries. And Oreos. "I put the healthy food in front of them, but they refuse to eat it!"

It's true, you can't force kids to eat healthy foods, but if we give them the choice, they're going to choose salt, fat, and sugar over leafy greens because salt, fat, and sugar appeals to our deepest, primal cravings stretching back to our caveman days when carbs were hard to come by. You had to fight tooth and nail for a little fat. And I agree: bacon tastes better than kale. But if you don't introduce bacon, burgers, and mocha-whipped-cream-frappuccinos to start with, sautéed spinach with a little butter and salt isn't bad.

I remember when my wife and I discovered that our son, Hank, had a massive sweet tooth (though he barely had teeth yet). Hank was two. It was his first Halloween. The look on his face when he bit into that Reese's Peanut Butter Cup was pure, unadulterated nirvana. When you eat sugar, yeast grows in your gut. The more sugar you eat, the more that wad of yeast expands, ramping up the sugar cravings. The yeast monster demands to be fed and parents have trouble saying no, especially when kids cry and stomp their feet. To avoid a battle in the first place, best not to introduce the mouth-watering junk.

In the West, we tend to stick with safe, non-threatening foods. Breakfast is really safe: pancakes, waffles, and cereal, the nutritional equivalent of a slice of cake. We rarely leave the bread and sugar comfort zone. I think we'd have fewer parents throwing up their hands and saying, "Hot dogs and spaghetti, that's all he eats!" if we stretched the comfort zone from an early age. In India, when babies are about 8 months old, they graduate to baby food with a little ceremony in which parents introduce curry for the first time, a little taste of the spice mixed with yogurt and ghee. In Japan, when babies have their first sushi rolls, there's a touch of wasabi on the rice; in Mexico, babies still in the mushy food stage get a little chili and lime mashed together with avocado; in Korea, parents warm up their babies palates with a smidge of kimchi and by their first birthday, they're accustomed to the spice. All over the world, babies' palates are gently being expanded, and by the time they're toddlers the new flavors are more familiar and easier to accept and you can avoid bland-white-food syndrome.

In the process of shooting *Daily Bread*, I've found that the story of hunger and obesity isn't always a story of haves vs. have-nots. They're often two sides of the same coin: the underfed and the overweight have the same problem; they don't have access to nutritious food. In fact, many of the places that struggled with hunger and malnutrition a generation ago are now seeing soaring rates of obesity.

The change has been so fast that we've been caught off guard. The UN is still focused primarily on hunger. Chronic undernourishment defined by calorie intake. Focusing on calories rather than a lack of nutrients misses the point. Calorie count has nothing to do with food quality.

There's an old adage, *"The hand that stirs the pot rules the world."* When the hand stirring the pot is more interested in profit than in our well-being, it's time we insist on healthier options and whenever possible, stir our own pots!

Daily Bread

Bee Wilson

Have you ever been in the supermarket and happened to pick up a shopping list that someone left behind? In the random scribbled food items, you seem to glimpse an entire way of life. You wonder what kind of person would eat "peaches, almond milk, corned beef, mayonnaise."

If you share my fascination at glimpsing what people eat behind closed doors, you will love this book. In *Daily Bread*, Gregg Segal has created an extraordinary set of portraits of children from around the world surrounded by the meals and snacks they consume in the course of a single week. I found myself enthralled by each image, trying to picture how all the ingredients fit together as part of the child's daily life. 8-year-old Frank from Senegal eats carrot salad and stew, heaps of fish and shrimp, white rice and baguettes, chocolate marble cake and Nutella chocolate spread. I wondered how Frank eats his Nutella. Does he spread it on a baguette? Or eat it by the spoonful?

These mesmerizing photographs show a generation of children learning to eat in a world of radical change. In Kuala Lumpur, the capital of Malaysia, 8-year-old Beryl eats fresh dragon fruit and pineapple cut into pretty shapes and wholesome home-made soups made with seaweed, fish, tofu, and greens; she also eats Kentucky fried chicken, chocolate cookies, and packaged cream crackers. Much of what Beryl is eating is classic Malaysian home cooking, but novel Western snacks are creeping in around the edges.

We sometimes talk as if healthy eating were an all-or-nothing game. Newspaper articles about obesity are often accompanied by simplistic photos showing vast mountains of greasy fast food hamburgers, fries, and ketchup, as if to imply that no obese person ever ate a vegetable. The truth about modern food is altogether messier, as these illuminating pictures confirm. In *Daily Bread*, Segal has created visual proof of the inconsistency of modern humans when it comes to eating—not least when those humans are children. Ten-year-old Cooper from Altadena, California, a dapper boy in a jacket and bow tie, enjoys sushi and salads and salmon with edamame beans. But he also eats large burgers and fries and pizza and chocolate chip pancakes with a sizeable pat of butter. When it comes to healthy eating, the important question is not whether we deny ourselves all foods high in sugar and trans fat, but where the balance of our diet falls.

The balance of what most children eat now is dramatically tipping away from homemade stews and vegetables and towards ultra-processed packaged foods and myriad snackfoods, many of them specially designed to appeal to children, such as the Milo chocolate milk which is drunk by children everywhere from Hamburg to Kuala Lumpur.

Across the globe, eaters are going through a "nutrition transition." Populations that once lived on lentils, starchy roots, and coarse grains are being replaced by more affluent and busy people with a taste for convenience foods, sliced white bread, and meat. This transition is written on our bodies, in the form of obesity, type 2 diabetes, tooth decay, and heart disease.

In a way, this transition is something to celebrate, because it signals the waning of acute hunger. None of the children featured in the photographs looks malnourished. Modern food distribution and rising incomes have given millions of people access to healthy foods such as fresh fruit for the first time. From California to Mumbai to Senegal, these children are enjoying melon and apples, grapes and oranges. Watermelon, which looks like a childish pink smile, seems to be a near-universal favorite for modern children, along with Cavendish bananas, which are currently the tenth most consumed food of any kind on the planet.

But if middle-class affluence buys fruit, it also brings sugary breakfast cereals and candy and a decline in the amount of vegetables children consume. One of the big surprises here is that, assuming there is enough to eat, the best quality diets are often eaten not by the richest but the poorest. In Segal's photographs, we can watch the food transition vividly playing out, child by child. Consider Anchal and Adveeta, two 10 year-old girls from Mumbai in India. Anchal lives with her family in an 8 by 8-foot aluminium hut. Her father earns under $5 a day and her diet includes no fresh fruit, yet she eats an appealingly wholesome and traditional diet of okra curries and lentils and flatbreads which Anchal's mother cooks from scratch each day on a single kerosene burner. Adveeta lives just a block away from Anchal but her parents are both scientists and she eats very differently. Her family's extra income buys Adveeta treats such as sweetened yogurt drinks and candy bars and fried snacks.

The same story is playing out all over the world, often with the same branded foods marketed by the same multinational corporations. The children featured here have totally distinct personalities and diverse hobbies yet they are often eating in eerily similar ways. Compare the diets of Paulo, age 9, from Sicily and Isaiah, age 16, in Long Beach California. In the past, a Sicilian boy would have grown up eating wildly different foods from his counterpart in the US, but now, their diets are converging. Both Paulo and Isaiah eat French fries and burgers; pasta and white bread. It's as if the boys' parents have been shopping at the same global superstore, even continents apart.

This project gives a human face to the problems of modern food. What these portraits reveal louder than words is that the food a child eats becomes an intimate part of his or her life. This is why it is going to be such a battle to persuade populations to change what they eat for the better. As Segal writes, we desperately need to move the needle on diet, but the obstacles to improving our eating are emotional as well as economic and social. Giving up a beloved food can feel like giving up part of yourself. I never felt this as strongly as I did when looking at these haunting and humorous photographs. In Kuala Lumpur, a 7-year-old girl is encircled by doughnuts and potato chips. She is hugging a giant bag of Big Bang seaweed snacks, holding it as tenaciously as a baby with a pacifier.

Amelia Torrisi, 12

Trecastagni, Sicily, Italy.
Photographed August 23, 2017 in Catania.

Amelia is from Trecastagni ("three chestnut trees"), an old Sicilian village in the hills below Mount Etna, an active volcano that erupted again last spring. She lives with her mother (an actress), her father (a masseur), and her 5-year-old sister in a house with a little vegetable garden where they grow tomatoes, bell peppers, and eggplants. The soil is very fertile from the volcanic ash, which has minerals that help plants thrive. Amelia eats mostly fresh fruits and vegetables and once a week some meat or fish. They rarely eat out; most everything is homemade and Amelia helps prepare meals like pasta with vegetables. Sometimes, when she goes out with friends, she eats a sandwich, which she says is the only unhealthy part of her diet. Amelia loves to read and cherishes her books. She would like to study medicine and if she has enough money someday, she'll buy a grand piano and help her parents when they're old.

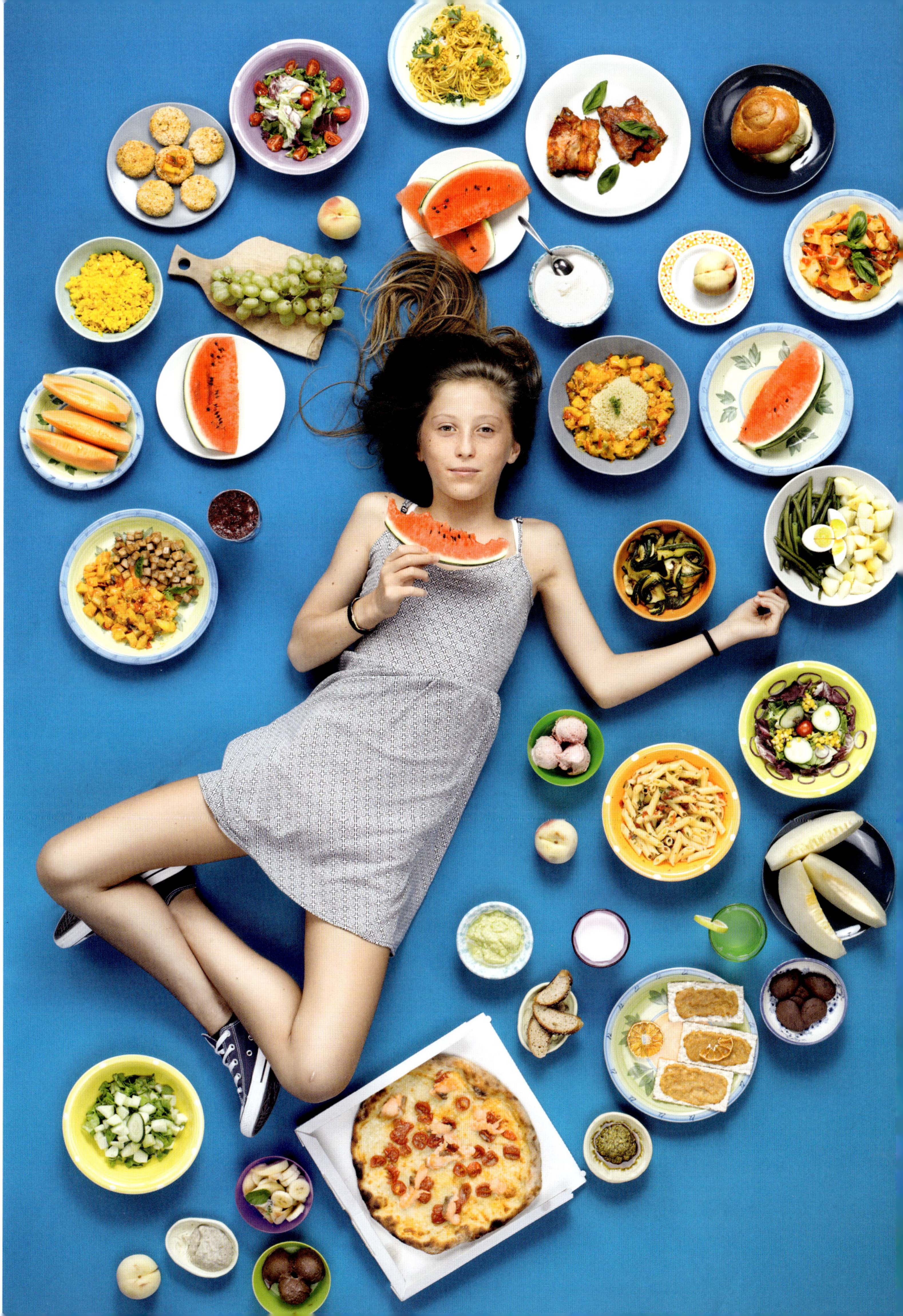

Thayla Reis Oliveira, 9

Brasília, Brazil.
Photographed August 19, 2018.

Thayla lives in a noisy, crowded neighborhood where music is played loud at all hours and soda cans and other trash litter the streets. Thayla's mom (a housekeeper) and dad (a gardener) struggle to make ends meet. Thayla studies at the Paranoá public school and in an afterschool program sponsored by the Ministry of Defense. Most poor kids in Brazil attend school to be able to eat, but the government has failed to provide adequate school lunches—little more than a glass of milk and a few crackers or a can of pre-cooked beans. Thayla would like to have more flavors in her diet and eat famous dishes of her country like feijoada (black beans with pork served with white rice, fried cassava flour, and sautéed collard greens). The army helps provide more substantial meals and bolsters the school curriculum, offering sports, recreation, crafts, English class, and civil studies. Thayla looks forward to playing tag and practicing capoeira at the army club. She sleeps with a cloth doll her mother had played with when she was a child. It has long blonde hair and nice clothes. If she had enough money, Thayla would buy clothes for the street kids who are worse off than her. Someday, she'd like to be a teacher.

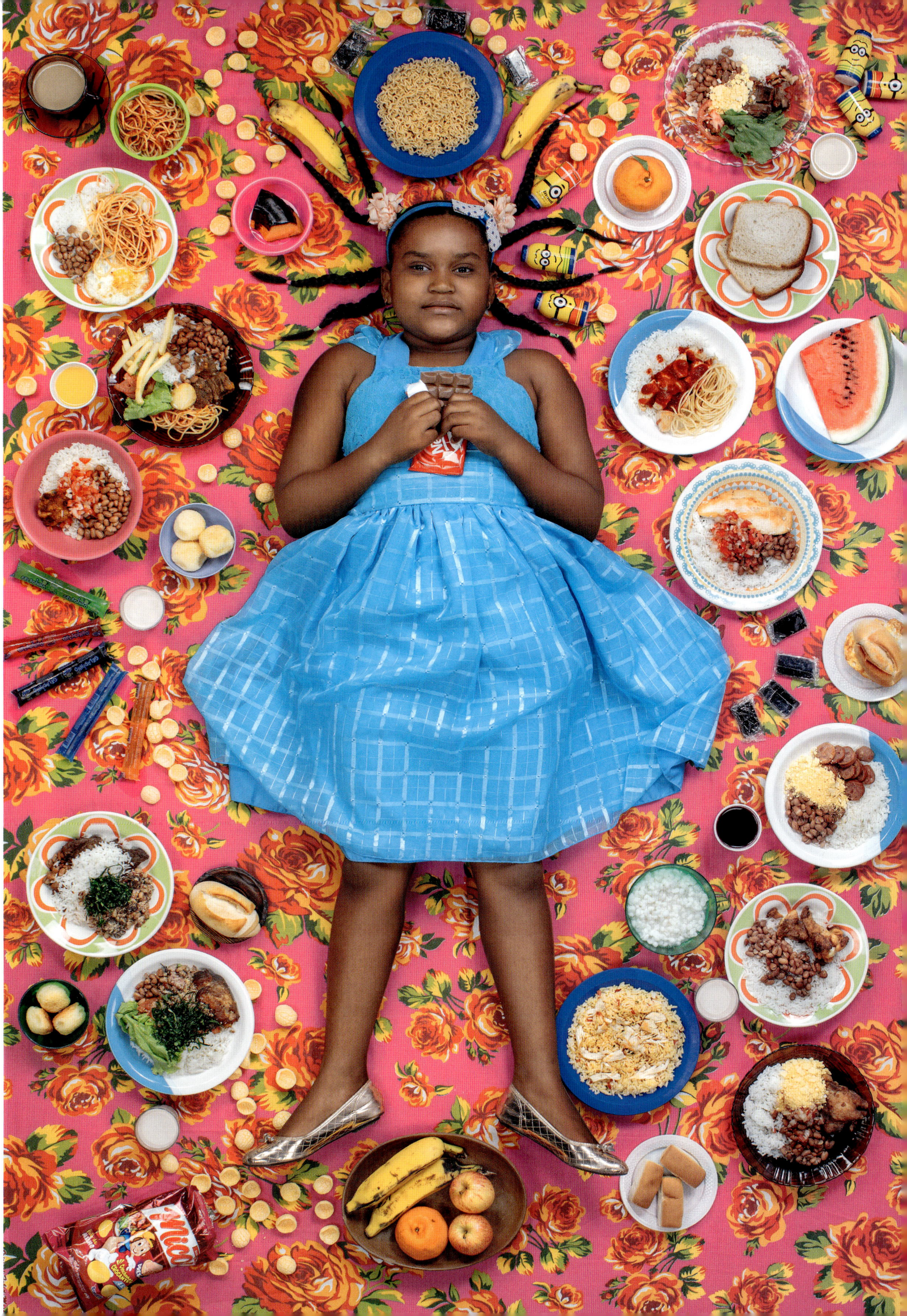

Cooper Norman, 12

Altadena, CA, USA.
Photographed January 30, 2016.

Cooper lives in the foothills of Altadena, California with his mom, a school administrator and dad, a human resources manager. Other than the cries of wild parrots and peacocks, his neighborhood is quiet, peaceful, and untraveled. At age 4, Cooper began taking karate classes and at 5, he took up classical guitar. He got into bow ties, too, which he wears for his guitar recitals. Cooper last wore this suit to a wedding in Palm Springs. The bride's uncle was so impressed with Cooper's table manners that he invited him out for dim sum. At Odyssey Charter School, Cooper plants all sorts of fruits and vegetables. He thinks of himself as an adventurous eater, willing to try almost anything, though Thai food (his mother's home country) is his favorite. His earliest memory of food is eating Cheerios in his stroller. Cooper plans to be a neurosurgeon when he grows up and, if he has enough money, will buy a teleporter, so he can visit his family in Thailand more often.

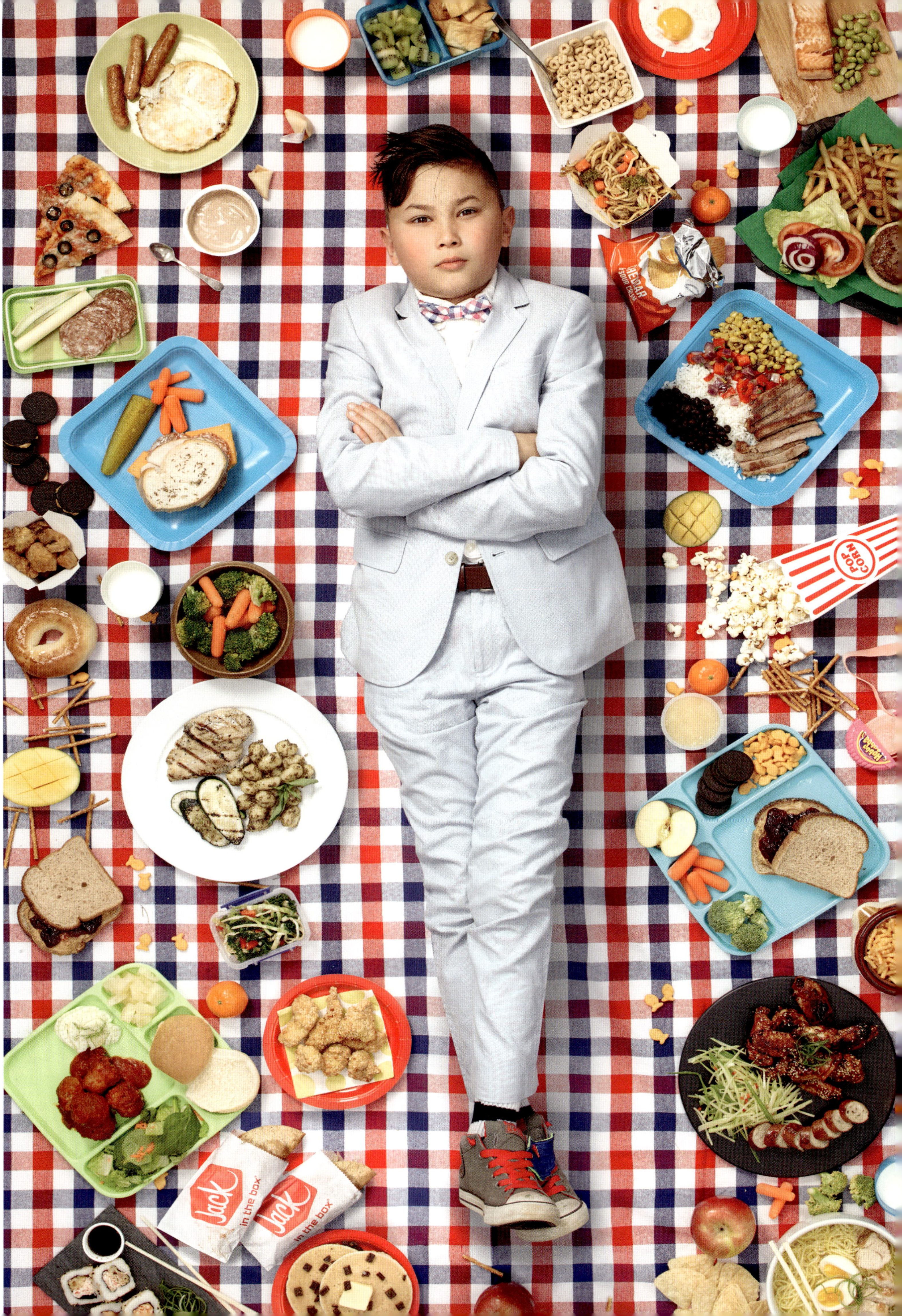
POP CORN
Jack in the box
Jack in the box

Nur Zahra Alya Nabila Binti Mustakim, 7

Kajang, Malaysia.
Photographed March 24, 2017 in Kuala Lumpur.

Nur's parents come from a rural village in East Malaysia. Her granny has supernatural beliefs passed down from long ago. She prepares food for the spirits and asks that they guard her family. Both Nur's parents work in the hospitality industry and have a three-bedroom townhouse in Taman Sinaran, Balakong, a busy neighborhood in the state of Kajang, south of Kuala Lumpur. People from different races live on Nur's street and they always greet one other and get together on weekends. Nur's diet includes a variety of Chinese, Indian, and Malay dishes like chee cheong fun, rice noodle rolls filled with steamed tofu, beancurd skin and fish balls served with a little sweet chili paste; roti canai, a flatbread eaten with dal and curry; and nasi lemak, a blend of rice, boiled eggs, cucumber, ancovies, peanuts and sambal (hot sauce) cooked in coconut milk and wrapped in banana leaves. 90% of Nur's meals are homemade; she loves her mother's cooking, especially her nasa ayam (chicken and rice), and her nasi lemak, which is mild and doesn't give her a stomachache like the spicy store-bought ones. The unhealthiest food Nur eats are the snacks and sweet drinks she buys at her school canteen. Nur is a tough, stoic girl; she doesn't cry when she falls off her bike. She just gets back on and keeps riding, setting an example for her two little sisters. When she grows up, Nur would like to be a dentist and help people take care of their teeth.

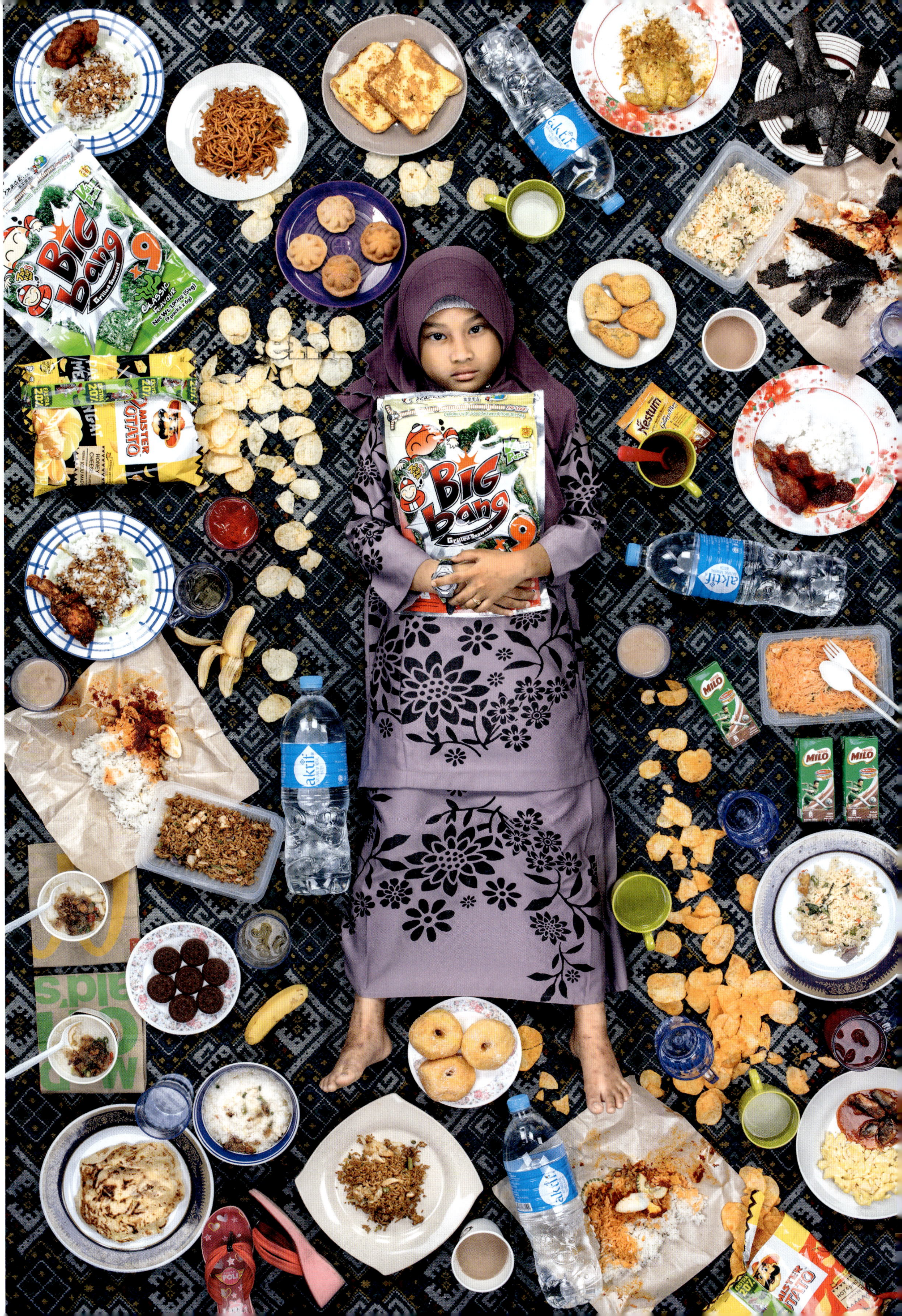
BIG Bang
Grilled Seaweed
aktif
MILO
MISTER POTATO

Chetan Menge, 10

Deonar, India.
Photographed March 12, 2017.

Chetan and his family of four live in a one-room flat in Deonar, a village outside Mumbai. Chetan's dad is a night watchman and his mom owns a beauty parlor. The family eats their meals in front of the little TV that is the centerpiece of their small home and when they're not talking about their favorite TV programs, they talk about their village and their farmhouse with its beautiful banana orchards. They don't pray before meals but just bow down to the food on their plates and put their palms together in namaste. Usually, Chetan is not full when he is finished eating; he always wants a little more, especially dessert. Chetan's father scolds his son for three things: 1) making noise with his mouth when eating 2) playing drums on his mom's pots and pans and 3) for not sitting up straight when he is eating. Chetan used to hate onions, but now he crushes them with his hands and eats them raw with chicken. For fun, Chetan invents stories about comical characters to tell his friends. He confesses that he is sometimes mischievous and laughs out loud at his friend's mishaps. Recently, he traveled by train to another district with 100 rupees in his pocket. When a neighbor saw Chetan hanging out at a local food stall, he called his mother, who was furious and gave Chetan a good scolding. Chetan is known for being kind to animals. He misses his most beloved tomcat, Mannya, and another stray cat, both of whom died due to some unforeseen events. If he had more money, Chetan would give to the homeless and feed the poor. He wishes his mother did not have to work so hard. Chetan works at his studies and would like to be a rocket scientist like Abul Kalam Azad, India's former president.

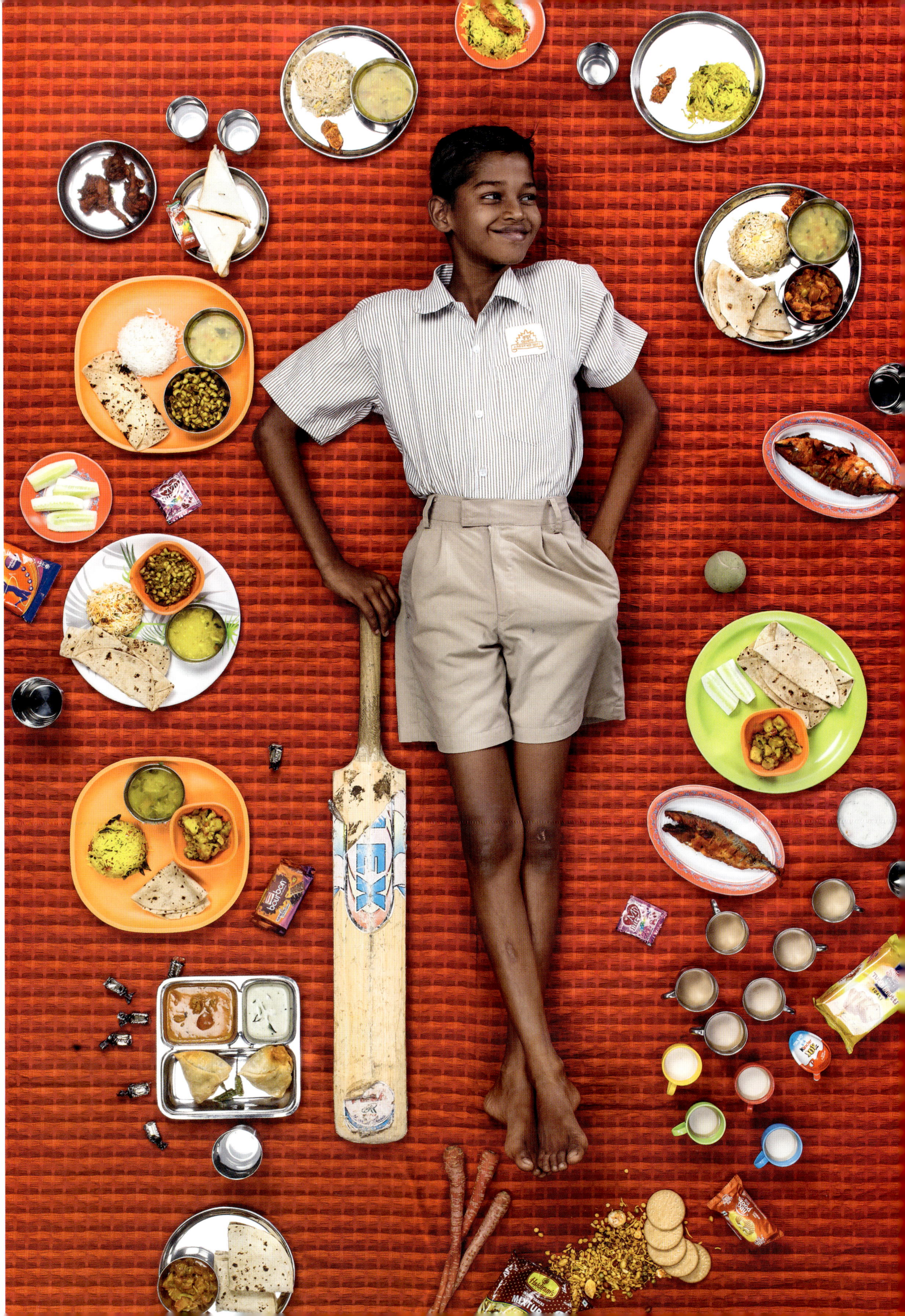
bourbon

Alexandra and Jessica Lewis, 9 and 8

Altadena, CA, USA.
Photographed February 21, 2016.

Alex and Jessica live in the foothills of Altadena with their daddy and papa who are engineers at the Jet Propulsion Laboratory, a NASA field center in La Cañada Flintridge, California. Their yard is filled with food: blackberry bushes, grape vines, and fruit trees—fig, peach, pomegranate, guava, mulberry, jujubes, and banana. They have chickens, too, and eat their eggs almost every day.

Jessica loves sweets and pizza with ham and is repelled by beans, peppers, sushi, and chocolate. She's good at drawing and daydreaming and on weekends the whole family rollerskates at Moonlight Rollerway. Jessica is the richest person on her street besides their neighbor Mary Anne. When she grows up, she wants to be an author and university professor.

Alex makes Hot Pockets, pizza rolls and quesadillas herself, but her favorite dish is macaroni and cheese. She refuses to eat Brussels sprouts or soggy leftover broccoli. She collects rocks and shells and is saving up for an Xbox 360 and Nintendo Switch. Alex makes people laugh without even trying because she's a spaz, she says. Her long-range goal is to get a PhD and have an outstanding career.

After the photo shoot, Alex and Jessica took much of the leftover food home to feed their chickens.

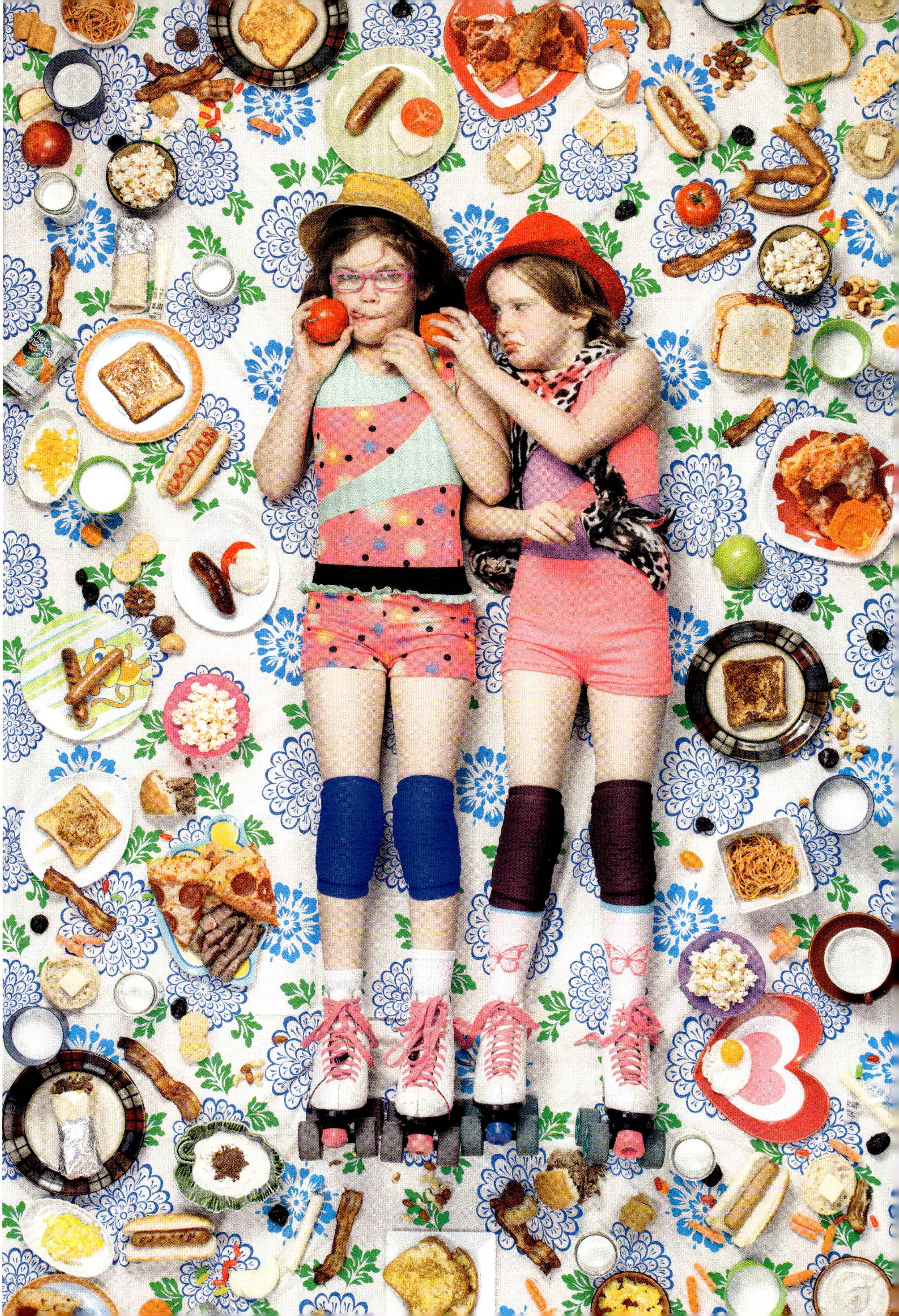

Iman Danial Azman, 11

Perak, Malaysia.
Photographed March 24, 2017 in Kuala Lumpur.

Danial is from the Telok Bakong district of Perak north of the capital, Kuala Lumpur. He lives with his two older siblings and parents in a kampung house, a traditional Malay dwelling built on stilts to avoid wild animals and floods. There is enough open green space for Danial to fly his drone and practice tricks like flips and figure 8s. Both of Danial's parents work for the Malaysian Ministry of Education. His mom came from a poor family but proved that you can study hard and become someone others respect. Though she has a demanding work schedule, Danial's mom finds time to prepare dinner most evenings. Danial is confident his diet is healthy because, "I make sure there is enough nutrition in my shakes." He noticed though, when looking at his portrait, that most of his food was brown: fried chicken, fried rice, fried fish, nasi lemak, cinnamon bread, Koko Krunch. Fried chicken, Danial confides, is his kryptonite. He's even learned to make fried chicken for himself, when he's hungry and his mother's at work. Since he was very young, Danial has tinkered with mechanical things. He'd like to be a motorcycle mechanic and can't wait to get his own bike. He's always checking the latest posts from Saiful Islam, a "motor blogger." Motorbikes are the last thing Danial thinks about before falling asleep.

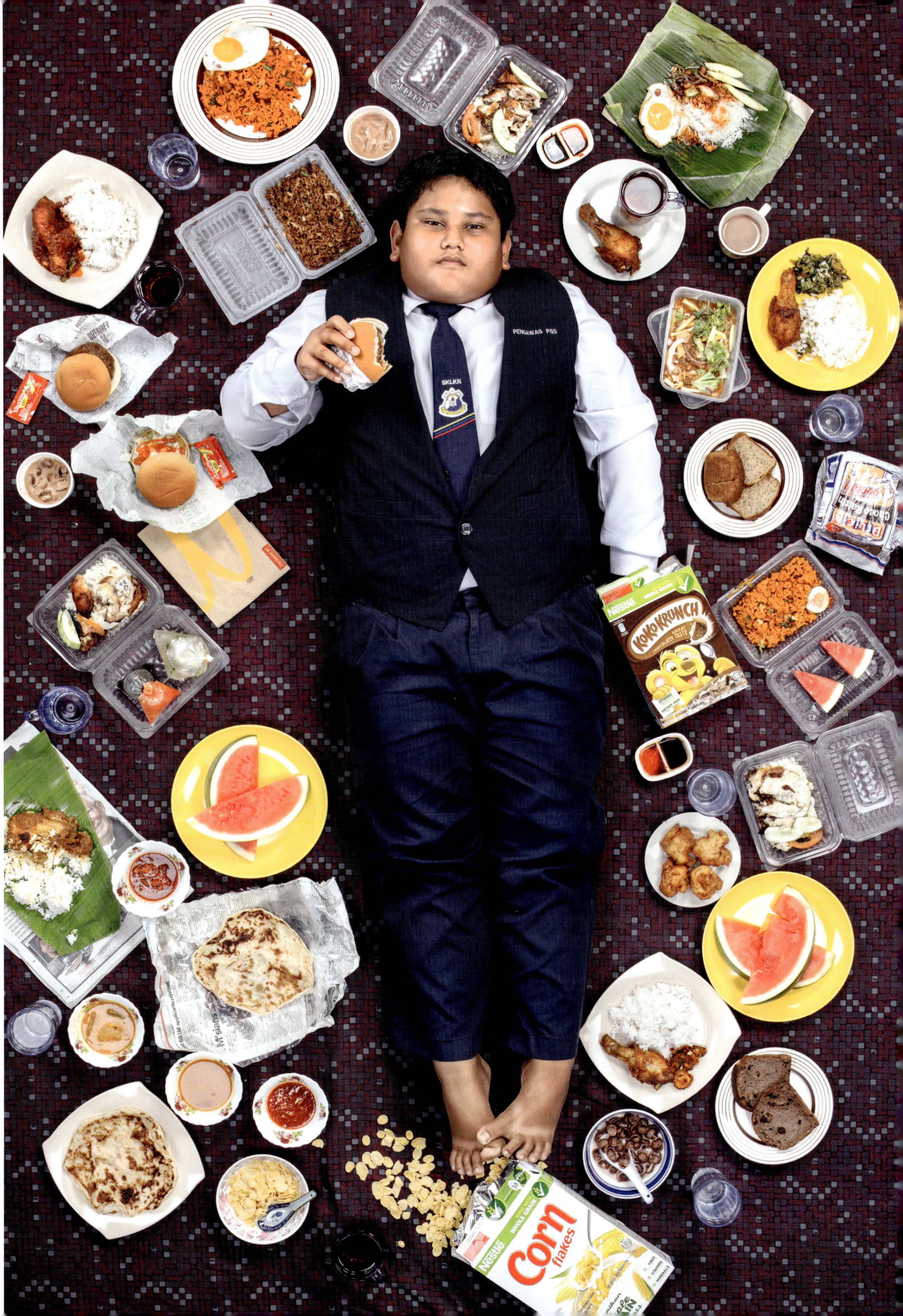
KOKO KRUNCH
Nestlé
Corn
flakes

Yusuf Abdullah Al Muhairi, 9

Dubai, UAE.
Photographed August 12, 2018.

Yusuf's mom came to Dubai from Ireland to work as a pastry chef and chocolatier. She married an Emerati man and they had one son before separating. Yusuf loves his mum's cooking though he makes scrambled eggs and toast all on his own. Yusuf likes to read, draw, climb, ride horses and create science projects. He thinks he'll either be a pilot or police officer when he grows up. If he had the money, he'd buy a Ferrari. His role models are Batman and his mother. Yusuf wishes for his mum to get married again and that he'll have brothers and sisters. Lying in bed at night, he thinks back to building a birdhouse with his granddad, fishing with him in the rivers in Ireland, and going to Warner Brothers Studio with his grandmom.

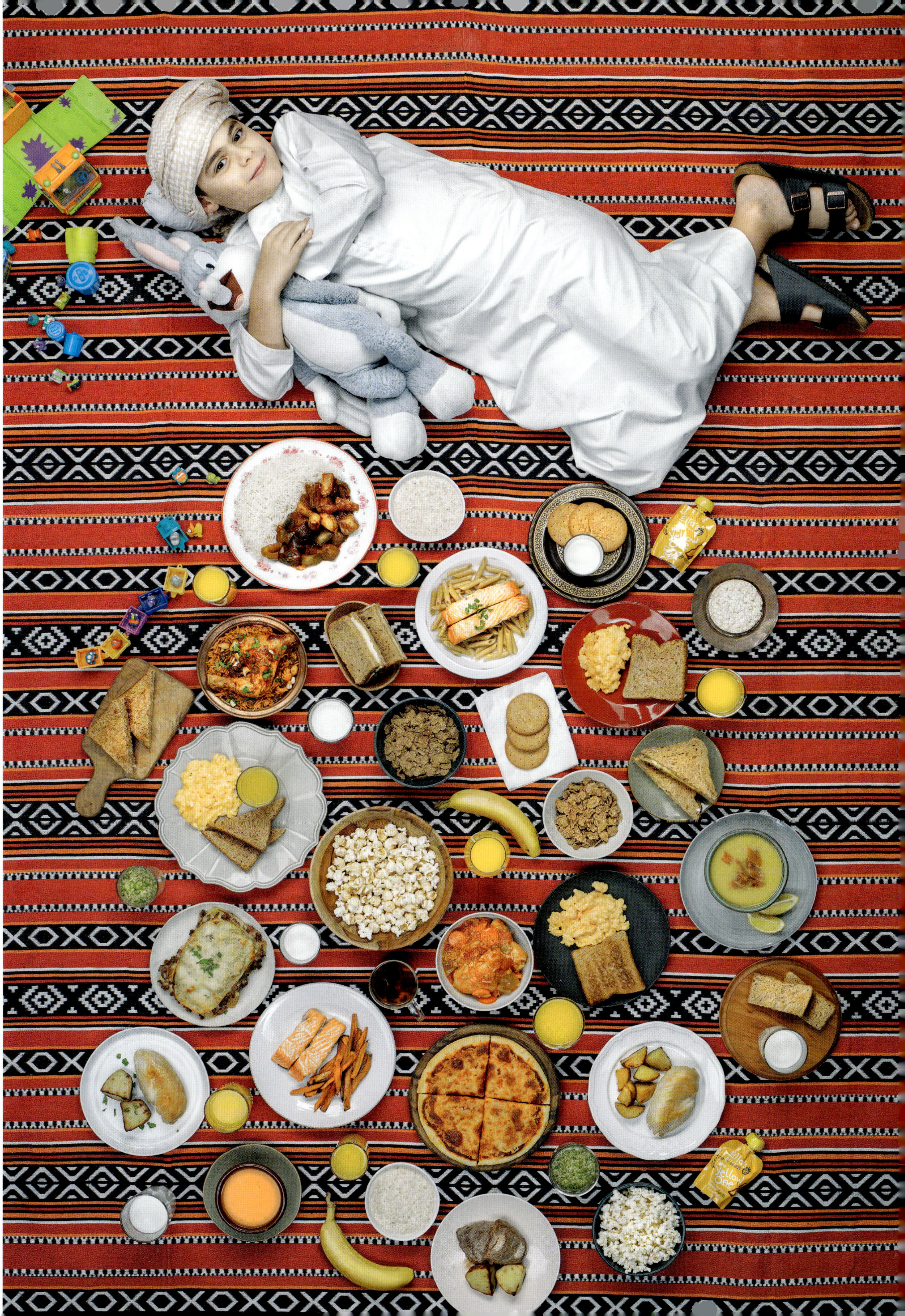

Greta Moeller, 7

Hamburg, Germany.
Photographed August 11, 2017.

Greta lives with her mother and younger sister in Hamburg, but spends quite a bit of time with her grandparents, too. On the path to her grandparents' home is a great big chestnut tree, and in autumn Greta searches in the foliage for chestnuts with her little sister. Greta's favorite food is fish sticks with mashed potatoes and applesauce. She can't stand rice pudding. One thing Greta is really good at is snapping her fingers, both hands at the same time. At night, while falling asleep, Greta thinks mostly about her mother, who is usually in the next room watching TV.

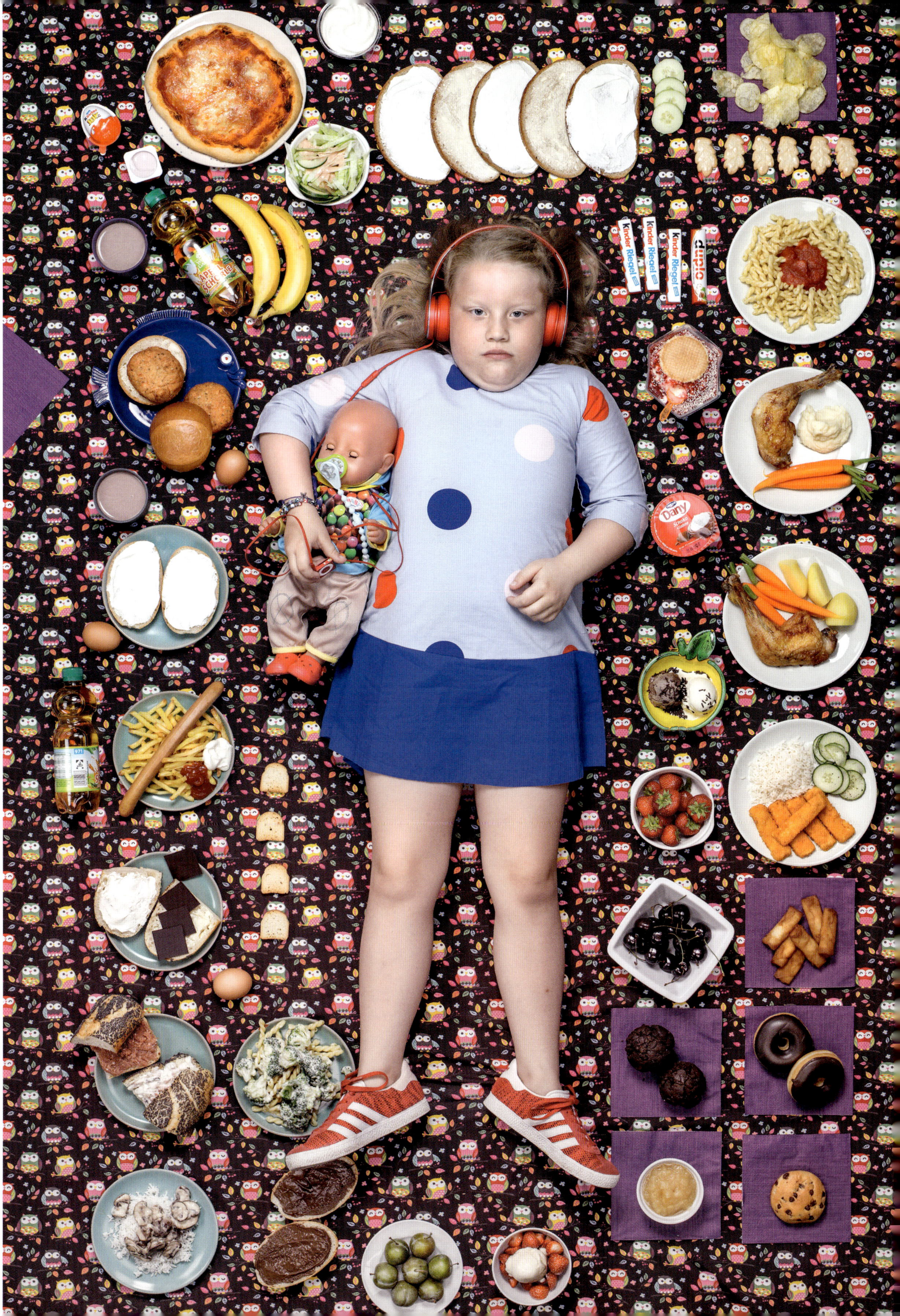

Kinder Riegel
Kinder Riegel
Kinder Riegel
Dany

Kawakanih Yawalapiti, 9

Upper Xingu region of Mato Grosso, Brazil.
Photographed August 19, 2018 in Brasilia.

Kawakanih is a member of the Yawalapiti tribe, one of fifteen Xingu tribes from the Amazonian Basin of Brazil. When she was born, Kawakanih's mother, Watatakalu, isolated her from those who didn't speak Arawaki, their native language. Only seven speakers of the language remained and her mother was afraid Arawaki would go extinct. In fact, Kawakanih is the first child to be raised speaking Arawaki since the 1940s and her mother says it's up to Kawakanih and her two siblings to keep the language alive. Kawakanih has also learned her father's dialect as well as Portuguese. She loves to read history books, especially ones about the Egyptians. Most of her days are spent playing in the river or helping with chores, like harvesting manioc (cassava), making tapioca, and fishing. Every couple of months, Kawakanih travels to Canarana for school where she learns computer skills, though no one in her village owns a computer; there is no electricity or running water. To get to the studio in Brasilia, Kawakanih and her mother traveled 31 hours from their village by boat, bus, and car. The red paint Kawakanih wears, traditionally made from ground urucum seeds, protects her from bad spirits and energy. A cluster of seed-pods are to the left of Kawakanih's head. Rainforest tribes have used the entire urucum plant as medicine for centuries. Kawakanih's diet is very simple, consisting mainly of fish, tapioca, fruit, and nuts. "It takes five minutes to catch dinner," says Kawakanih. "When you're hungry, you just go to the river with your net."

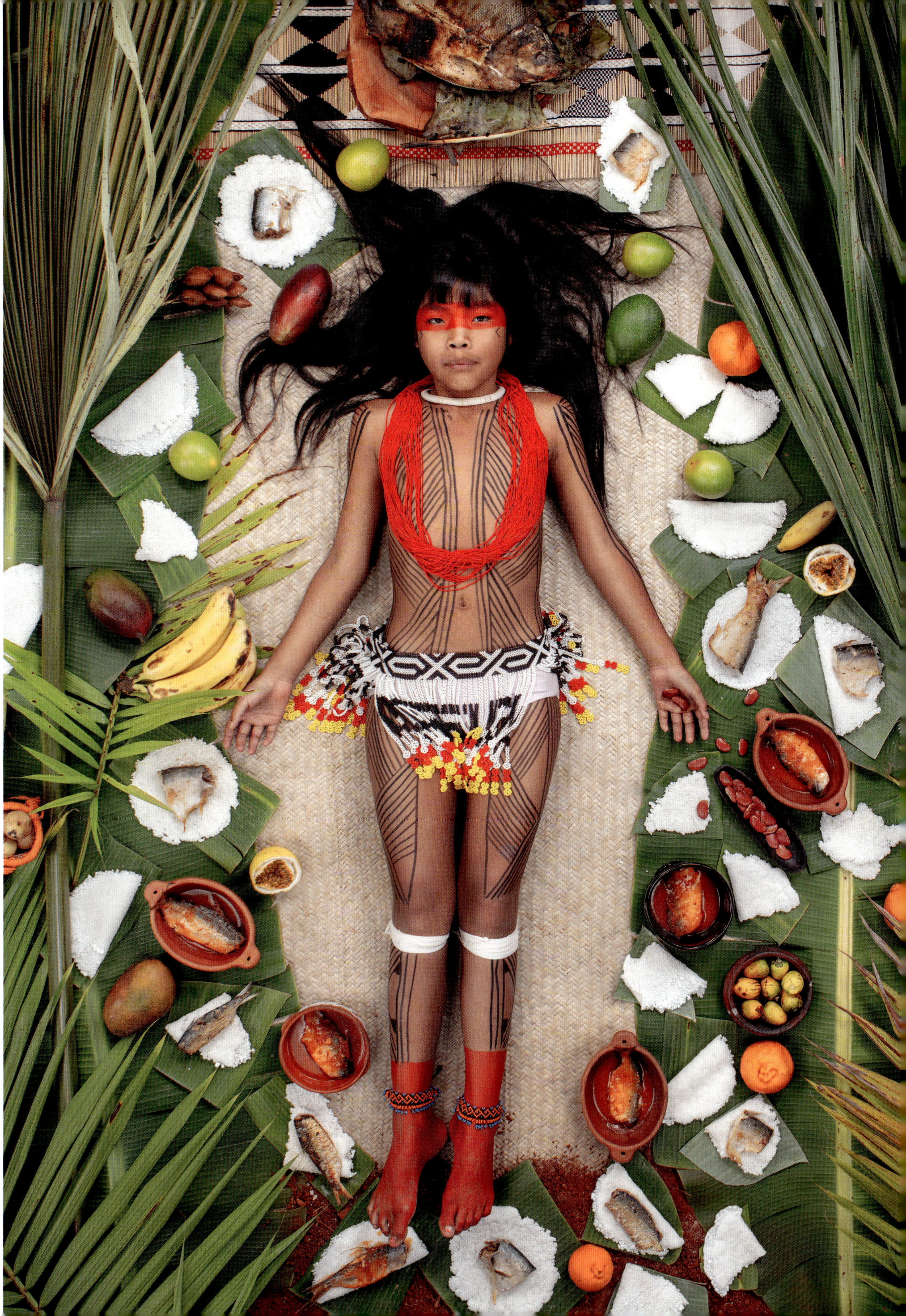

Henrico Valias Sant`anna de Souza Dantas, 10

Brasilia, Brazil.
Photographed August 18, 2018.

Henrico lives in a posh suburb of Brasilia with his mom, a film producer and advertising executive, and his two siblings. Henrico's mom, grandma, and maid do the day-to-day cooking, though Henrico likes to invent his own snacks. His favorite dish is feijoada, a Brazilian stew of black beans and pork, served with a side of white rice, farofa (fried cassava flour), and collard greens. Henrico likes dessert, too: chocolate soufflé; Toblerone and Talento bars; anything with Nutella; brigadeiro, a ball of baked condensed milk and chocolate; buttered toast sprinkled with Nescau powder, a treat his uncle invented; and one of his own creations—steak covered with sliced banana. Henrico has mastered video games like LittleBigPlanet, Lego Marvel, and Don't Escape 3. He listens to Justin Bieber, Maroon 5, and Gato Galactico, watches *Iron Fist* and *The Flash* on Netflix and is a Star Wars fan. From participating in Daily Bread, Henrico discovered that he eats a wide variety of food. He has no idea what he wants to do when he becomes an adult. There is nothing missing in his life. He is perfectly content.

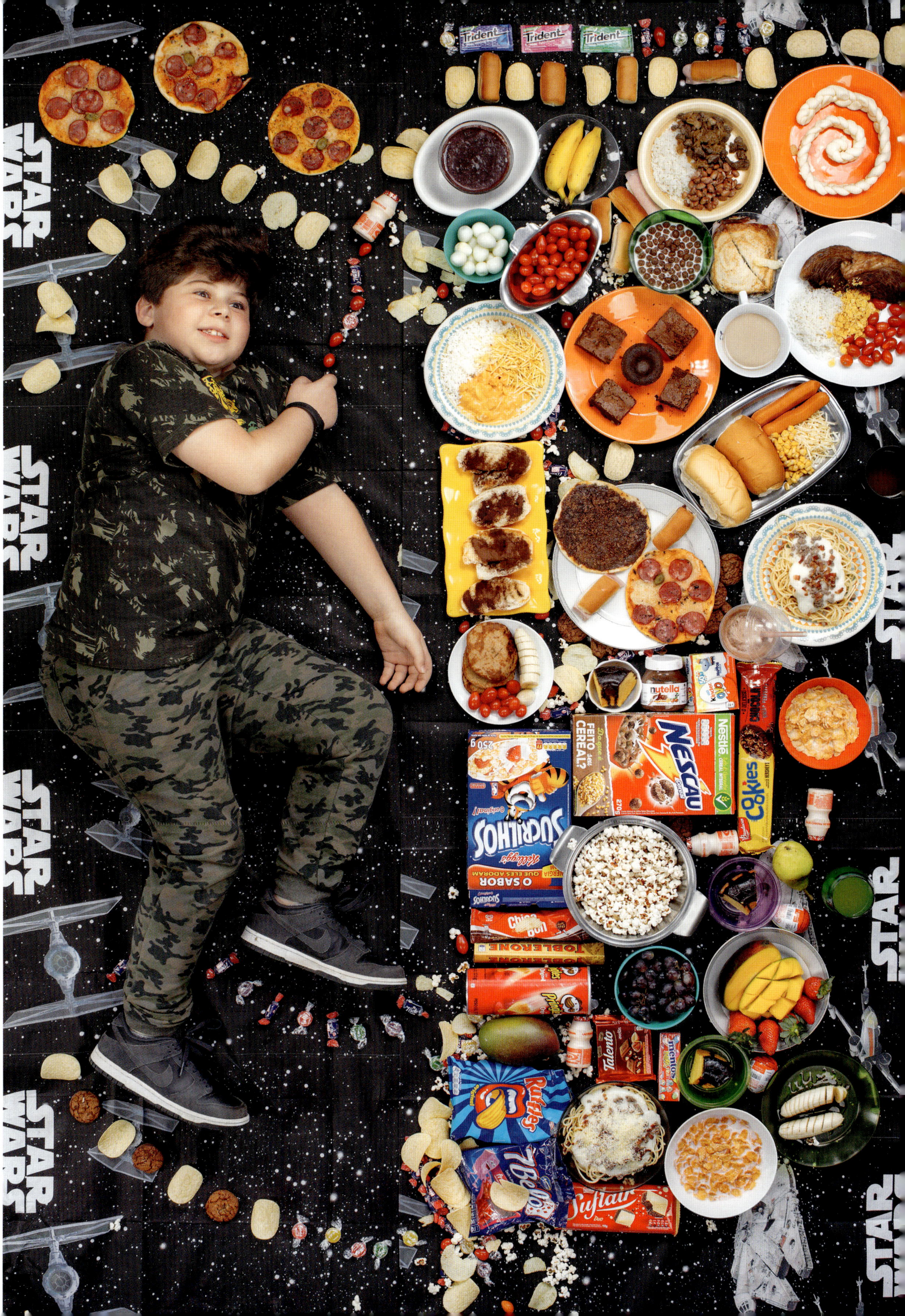
STAR WARS
Trident
Trident
Trident
nutella
NESCAU
Nestlé
FEITO COM CEREAL?
SUCRILHOS
Kellogg's
TOBLERONE
Pringles
Ruffles
Cookies
Talento
mentos
Suflair

Andrea Testa, 9

Catania, Sicily, Italy.
Photographed August 23, 2017.

Andrea lives in a single house surrounded by a little garden and lava stones with his parents and 6-year-old sister, Vittoria. Andrea's father is an officer in the Italian army and his mother is a housewife who does all the cooking. Andrea's favorite dish is pasta carbonara with plenty of bacon. He loves the scent of orange blossoms and cherries. He won't touch cauliflower. If he had enough money, Andrea would buy a drone and a little dog, which he would name Ettore (Hector). Andrea performs magic tricks for his family and friends. His hero is Robinson Crusoe. Andrea would like to be a doctor because they make a lot of money.

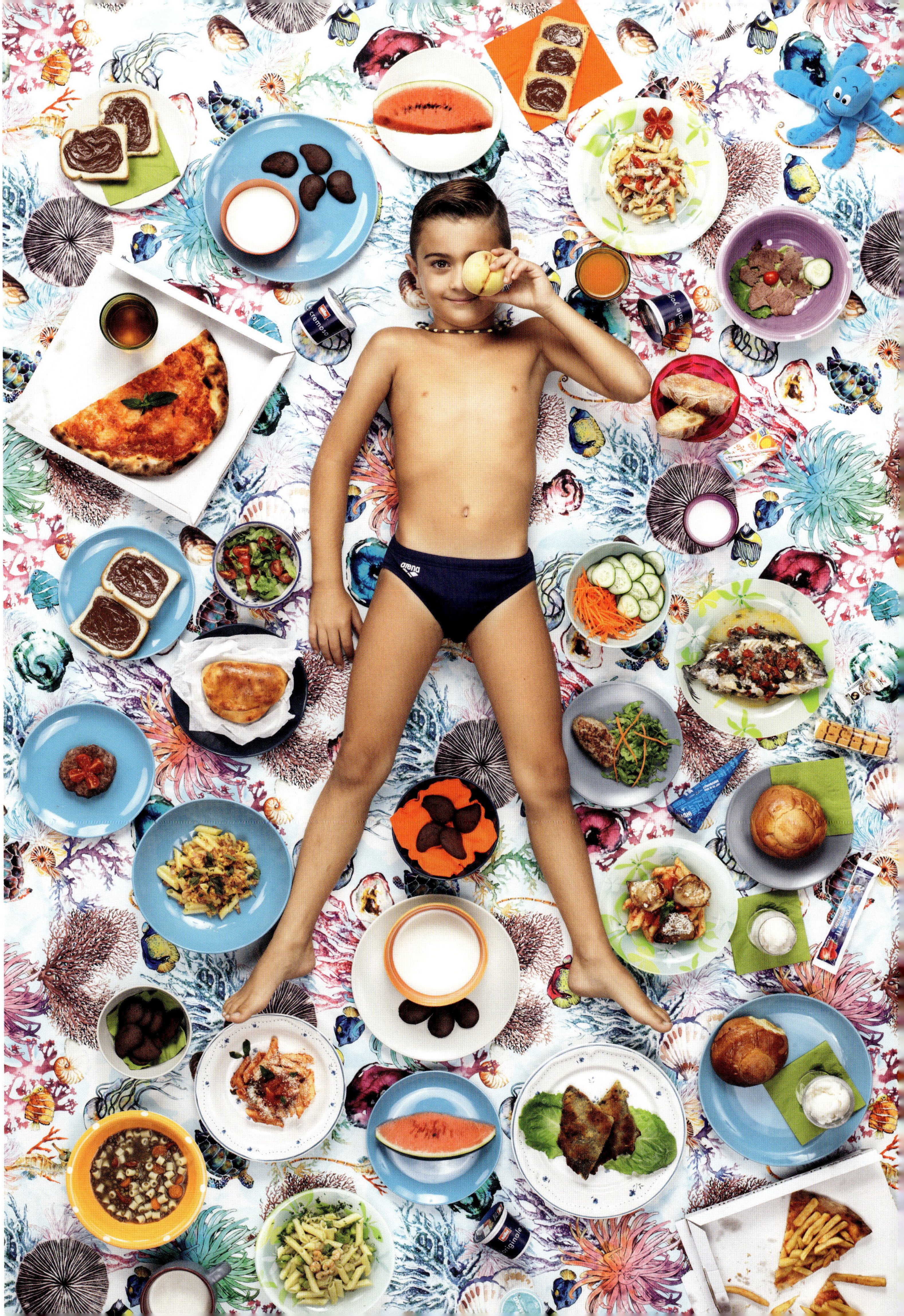

Adveeta Venkatesh, 10

Deonar, India.
Photographed March 11, 2017.

Adveeta, an only child, lives with her maternal granny—who prepares most of her meals—and her parents in a spacious flat with a balcony overlooking Deonar, a suburb of Mumbai. The air is often hazy from fires burning at Deonar Dumping Ground, India's oldest and largest landfill, an 18-story, 12-million-ton mountain of trash. Adveeta's mother and father are scientists at a government research center in Mumbai. They make it home in time for dinner. While at the table, no one uses gadgets or watches TV. Before eating, Adveeta says a prayer of gratitude for the food on her plate. A vegetarian, she loves South Indian cuisine, particularly dosas (pancakes made from fermented rice and lentils) served with spicy chutney and yogurt. A few years ago, Adveeta was a picky eater. She didn't eat 99% of the food she eats now. But as her father discovered during the photo shoot, she's also eating more snacks and sweets. "I can't believe Adveeta is eating all that junk!" he commented, as the pictures popped up on my monitor. "I'm going to have to have a talk with her mother!" Adveeta studies drama, performs classical Indian dance, and prefers to solve puzzles and riddles than to play with Barbie dolls. She's only cried once in the last year. While traveling in Jakarta and Bali, she contracted chicken pox and was kept isolated from her cousins. Adveeta plans to be a veterinarian and to contribute extra money to orphanages and animal shelters.

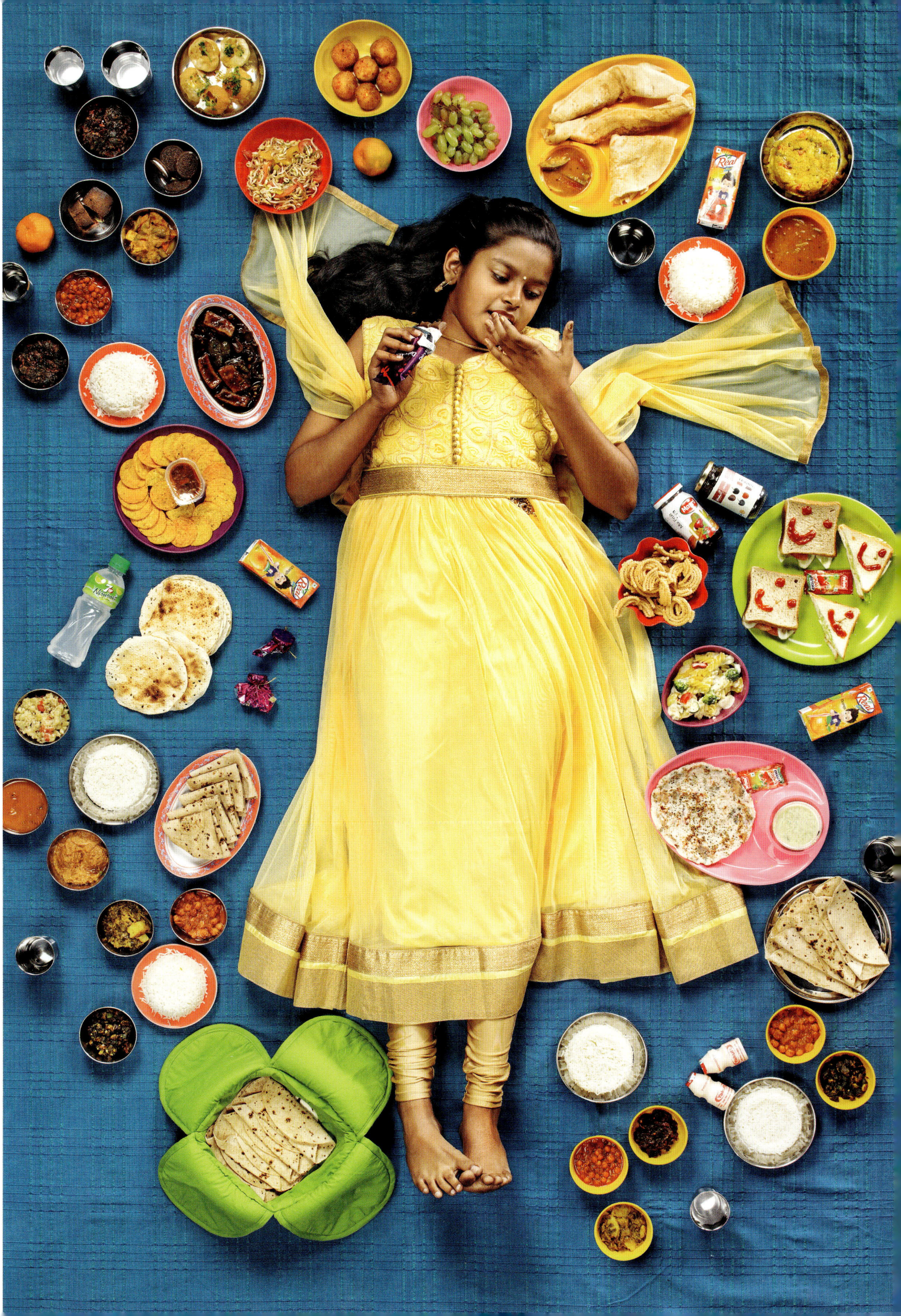

Meissa Ndiaye, 11

Dakar, Senegal.
Photographed August 30, 2017.

Meissa shares a single room with his dad, mum, and brother in the heart of Parcelles Assainies, which means "sanitized plots." A treeless, sandy region of Dakar, Parcelles Assainies was developed in the 1970s to house the poor overflowing from the city. Meissa lives opposite the futbol stadium and open-air market, hundreds of stalls selling everything from fresh fish to wedding dresses. In late August, tethered goats line the streets before Eid al-Adha, the Festival of the Sacrifice. Meissa, a devout Muslim and student at Quran school, loves goat meat and sweet foods like porridge, though in the week he kept a diary of his meals, he ate very little meat. More often, he filled up on French bread stuffed with spaghetti, peas, or fried potatoes. Meissa's mum and anties prepare his meals, though once or twice a week they get takeout. Meissa loves futbol most of all and hopes to be a star player like Messi or Ronaldo. If he had enough money, he'd buy a nice little sports car. He wishes his mum and dad, a refrigerator technician, could immigrate to France so that they can earn more money.

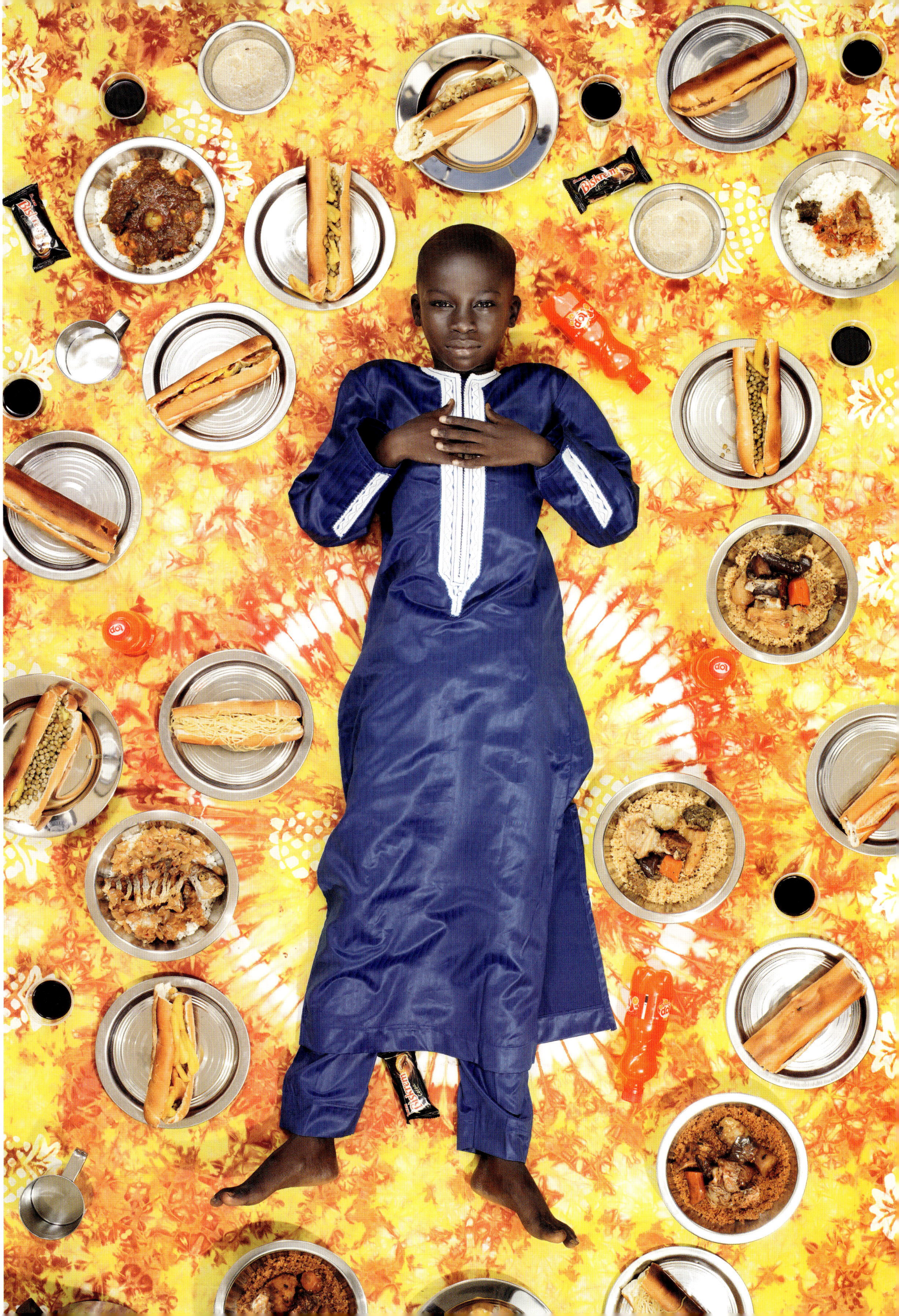
Biskrem

Asma and Fatima Ahmed Kindi, 10 and 7

Ajman, UAE.
Photographed August 12, 2018 in Dubai.

Asma and Fatima live with their parents and four siblings in a lively neighborhood of Ajman, an emirate south of Dubai. Their dad, whose muscles are as big as Arnold Schwarzenegger's, does security for movie productions and leads desert safaris for tourists. Mom runs the house. Asma and Fatima are not picky eaters—they eat everything except macaroni with béchamel sauce. They especially like pizza, chocolate, hot dogs, and Syrian kibbeh. They have never grown or harvested anything nor learned to prepare any foods. Asma would like to be an optometrist. Fatima would like to be a pediatrician. They'll have enough money to buy a villa, car, clothes, a home for mother, and a hospital for her, too, if she is sick. Asma and Fatima would like to be with their parents till the last day of their lives.

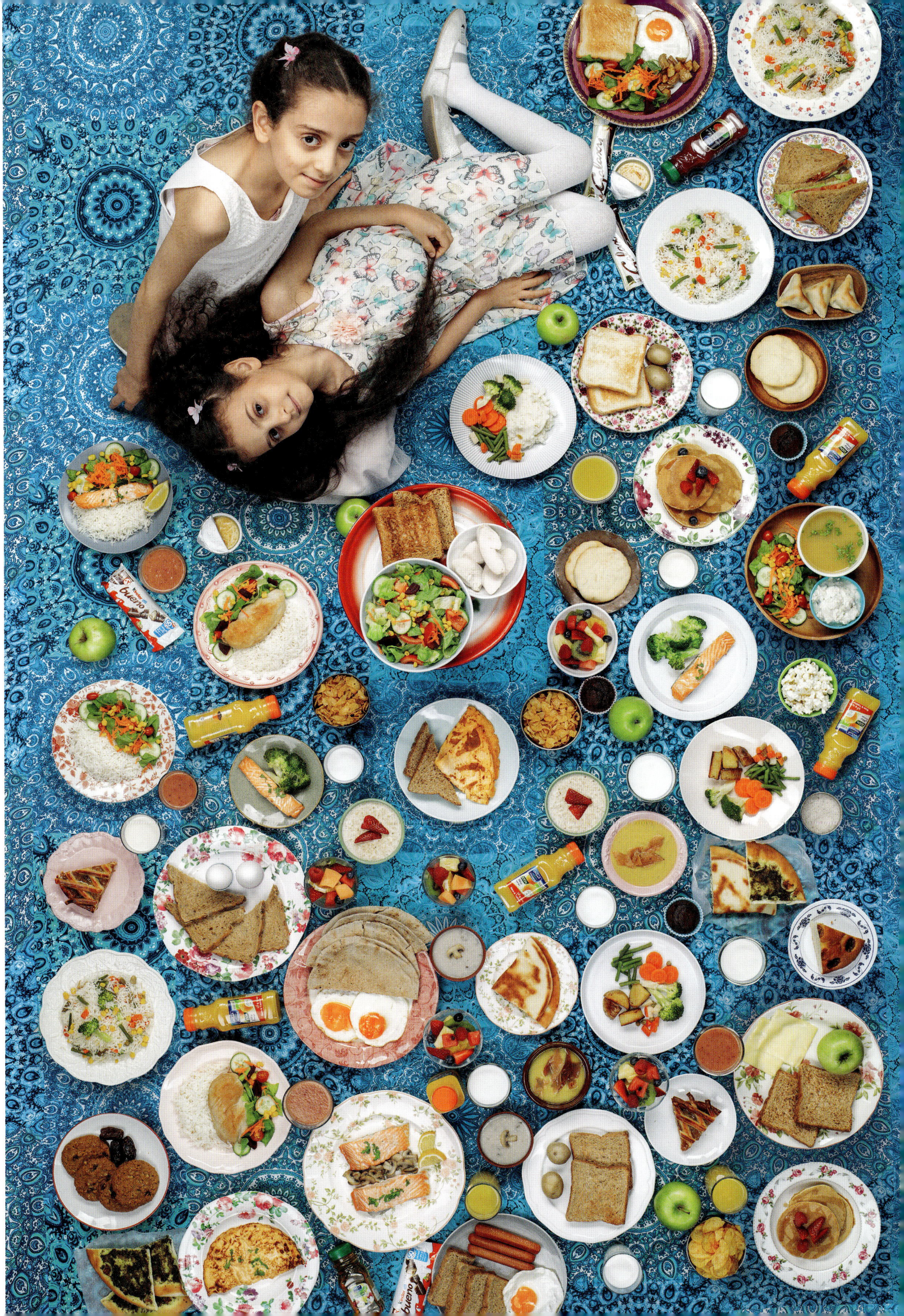
bueno

Davi Ribeiro de Jesus, 12

Brasilia, Brazil.
Photographed August 18, 2018.

Davi lives with his dad, step-mom, and three siblings in a tidy one-room house in the Santa Luzia favela, a slum at the edge of the largest garbage dump in Latin America. The space is filled by three beds, a sofa, TV, refrigerator, two wardrobes, a cooker, and a small table where they share their meals. A mosaic of mats and scraps of plywood cover the dirt floor. Davi has his own shelf where he arranges his clothes, his toy car collection, and his mobile. There's no garbage collection and the power goes down frequently. When it rains, scattered garbage turns to sludge and oozes into homes, but Jesus keeps Davi and his family safe and happy. They go to a church nearby every Saturday night and Sunday morning. Davi's dad is looking for work as a digger. He has his own pick, shovel, and grubber. Davi's step-mom handles the cooking. Davi will eat almost anything except bitter legumes though most days he has beans and rice, maybe with a little pork. He can cook fried eggs, porridge, and pasta for himself. Sometimes there are treats, like sweet popcorn. He never goes to bed hungry. Davi laughs easily and is crazy about kites. He and his friends, Maxwell, Junior, and Romário have kite fights in the favela's empty lots where bored stray dogs scratch at fleas or sniff around for food. Davi adopted five strays and gave them names: Lassie, Beethoven, Tchutchuquinha, Belinha, and Piloto. He also has a chicken and wants a horse. He wants to learn all about cars, motorcycles, helicopters, and guns, too. His dad taught him to drive and now he dreams of having a Chevy. He'd like to be a cop when he grows up because it's better to be a cop than a thief.

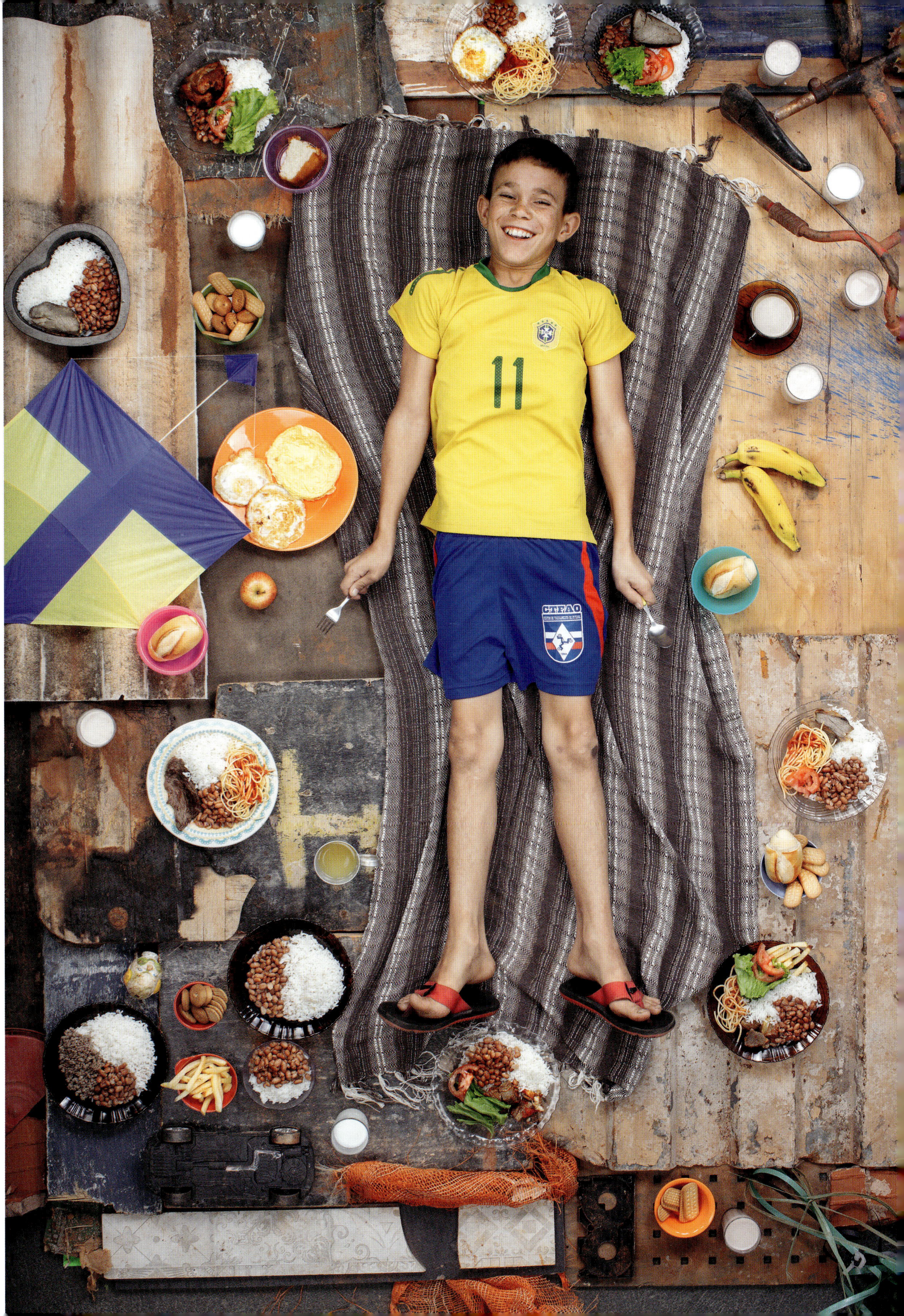
11
CEFAD

Beryl Oh Jynn, 9

Kuala Lumpur, Malaysia.
Photographed March 25, 2017.

Beryl lives in a quiet condominium with her parents and two brothers. She goes to S.J.K. Han Ming, a national Chinese school walking distance from home. Beryl's dad is an engineer and her mother runs a day care. Beryl's earliest memory of food is porridge and cake. Her favorite dish is spaghetti with carbonara sauce. Beryl grows bok choy and spinach in her balcony garden, is not permitted to drink sodas, and refuses to eat ginger. She would like to be a cheerleader.

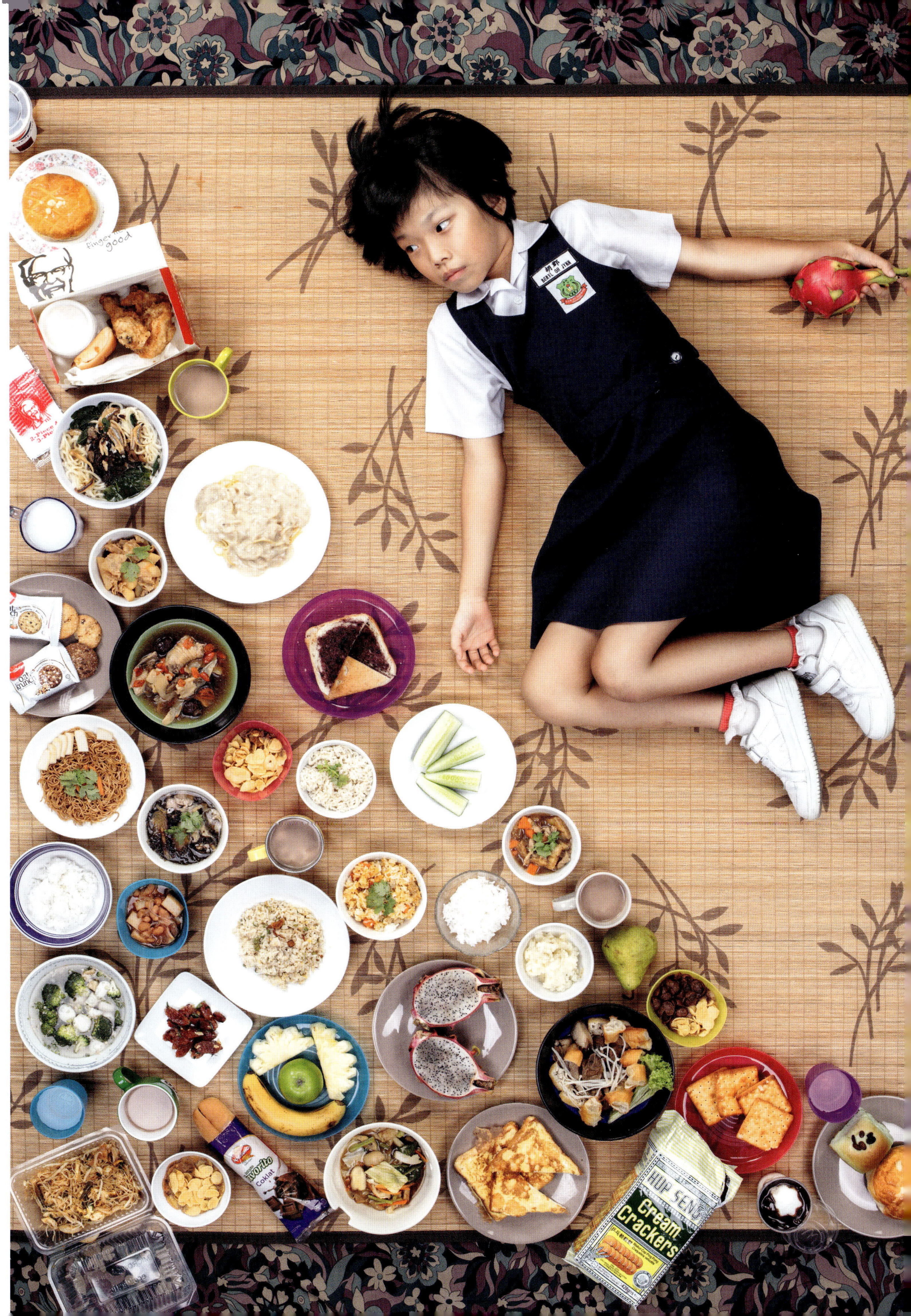
HUP SENG
Cream Crackers

Jesus Lino, 16

Los Angeles, CA, USA.
Photographed March 21, 2016.

Jesus was raised by his mom, who was a teenager when she left her family and home in Michoacan, Mexicio and made her way north to Los Angeles. Jesus, his mom, and his two older sisters shared a one-bedroom apartment south of Downtown infested with roaches and rodents. Jesus saw little of his dad whom they discovered had another family. The only meal Jesus ate most days was dinner. His one-hour commute to school didn't leave time for breakfast and the school lunch was so unappetizing, a piece of fruit was all he could stomach. Mom made chicken and rice most nights but on special occasions, she'd prepare Jesus' favorite: tamales with red chili sauce. Vegetables were absent from Jesus' diet; he just didn't care for them. Growing up, Jesus was aware there were people worse off than him. He'd see the homeless begging for cash and though some people warned him to keep his distance, he wanted to help. In high school, he joined a student organization to feed the homeless and volunteered with Peace Over Violence, a non-profit helping victims of domestic abuse. Jesus has always admired his mother's perseverance and optimism. She struggled to raise her family and make ends meet but was always upbeat, positive that God would bring good things. Jesus is now a sophomore at Harvard University with a double major of applied mathematics and psychology. He has had more opportunities than he could ever have imagined though knows there are obstacles ahead; he hasn't met anyone from his background who is very successful.

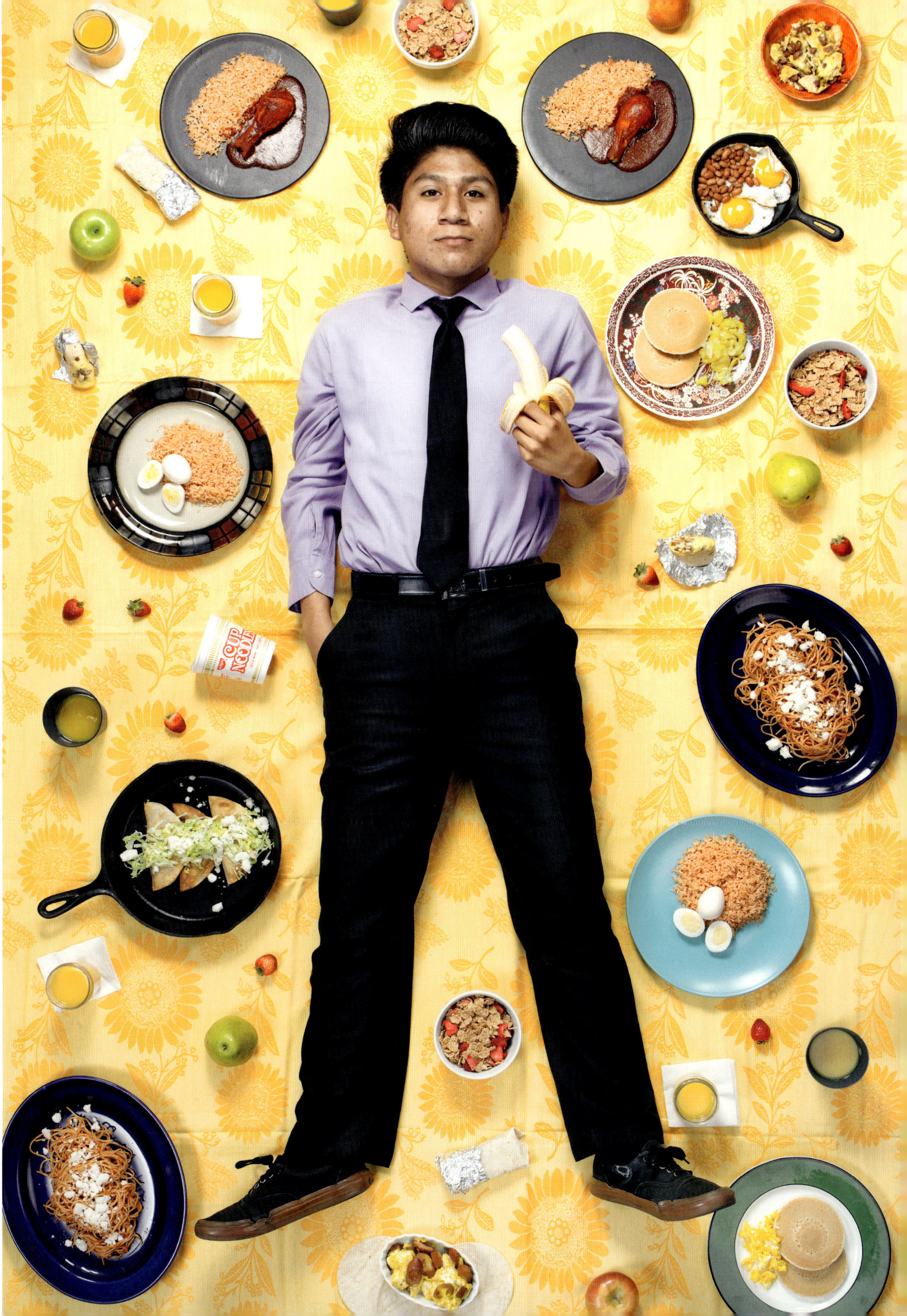
CUP

June Grosser, 8

Hamburg, Germany.
Photographed August 11, 2017.

June's mom is a fashion photographer, though she hasn't yet photographed her daughter. June must have observed her mother at work or she's just a natural model, completely assured in front of the camera. June can sing almost all the songs she hears on the radio—and dance to them. She has no role model. She intends to be her own role model. She'd like a dog, but her parents won't allow her. She figures if she can make enough money, she may be able to bribe her mother to get one. June's favorite food is schnitzel. She doesn't care for curry and truffles and didn't like broccoli either until recently. She is full after meals but hunger returns quickly. At dinner, June doesn't talk much, but rather listens to her parents discuss politics, elections, and what's going on in the world. The things she likes most about herself are her hair, her long eyelashes, and her imagination, her fantasies. One of her wishes is to fly to the moon, though she'd rather focus on wishes that will be fulfilled. June is reading *The Vampire Diaries* and as she's lying in bed at night trying to fall asleep, she often wonders if vampires really exist.

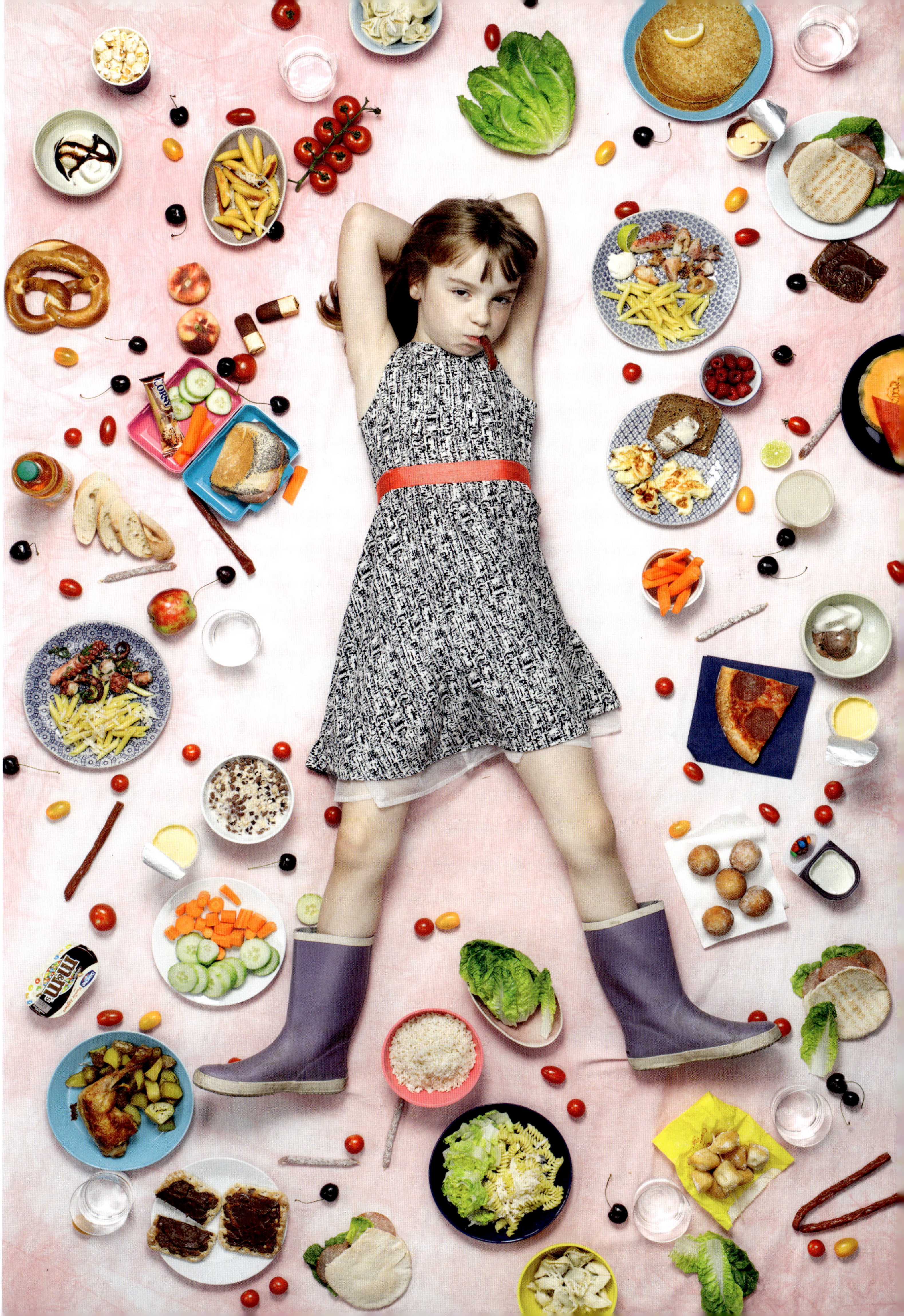
CORNY

Altaf Rabbal DLove Bin Roni, 6

Kampung Kerdas, Gombak, Malaysia.
Photographed March 26, 2017 in Kuala Lumpur.

Altaf and his family live in Kampung Kerdas, a small village of about 30 families on the outskirts of Kuala Lumpur. There are many children Altaf's age. They chase each other around the neighborhood almost every evening and pick fruit from the trees: mango, rambutan, and mangosteen. If it's raining, they'll play marbles. Often, Altaf visits his grandparents who live five minutes away. Altaf's father makes and sells satay sticks at his own stand and runs delivery for a Malaysian online platform part-time while Altaf's mom takes care of the house and kids; she's expecting her fourth soon. Altaf's favorite food is his father's chicken and beef satay. It's seasoned with ginger and herbs, roasted over a charcoal fire and served with sliced, cold cucumber. Altaf dips his satays in a tangy sauce made with roasted ground peanuts, chili paste, garlic, and lemongrass. Altaf will eat any "tasteful" food (made with a lot of ingredients and flavors) and likes raw, leafy greens like ulam-ulam, a salad eaten with anchovies, cincalok (a condiment made from fermented krill), and sambal (hot sauce). The only foods Altaf avoids are pickles and other sour things. Altaf collects parcel stickers, big, colorful ones, and likes to discover new things. He loves science because to him it is magic. When he grows up, he wants to be a pilot. He loves to fly like birds while watching the skies and clouds. As he falls asleep, Altaf thinks of what he'll do tomorrow: catch fish, climb a tall fruit tree, or cycle far from his village.

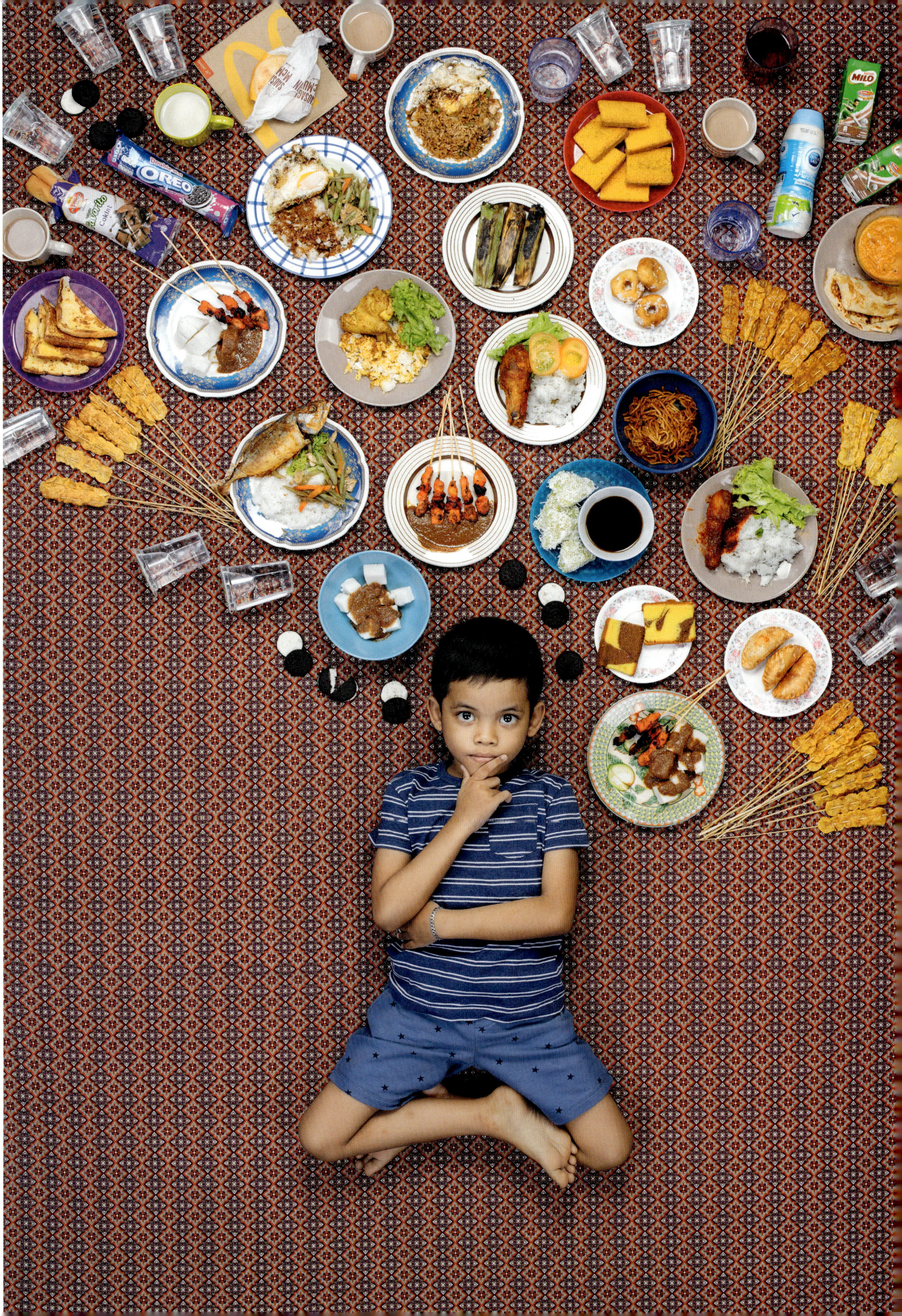
OREO
MILO

Rosalie Durand, 10

Nice, France.
Photographed August 18, 2017.

Since her parents split up, Rosalie has lived part time with her mom, and part time with her dad, which allows her to see both the sea and mountains from home. Rosalie's passions are Thai kickboxing, rock climbing, and gymnastics. She eats a healthy diet (which includes lots of fresh fish, like sardines) thanks in part to her father, a restaurateur, who has taught her to make crepes, salads, and lentils with sausage—her favorite dish.

Rosalie gets her sense of style from her mother, a fashion designer, and plans to be an interior designer. She notices she's getting older because she has a phone. There's nothing missing in Rosalie's life, though if she had enough money, she'd buy a yacht.

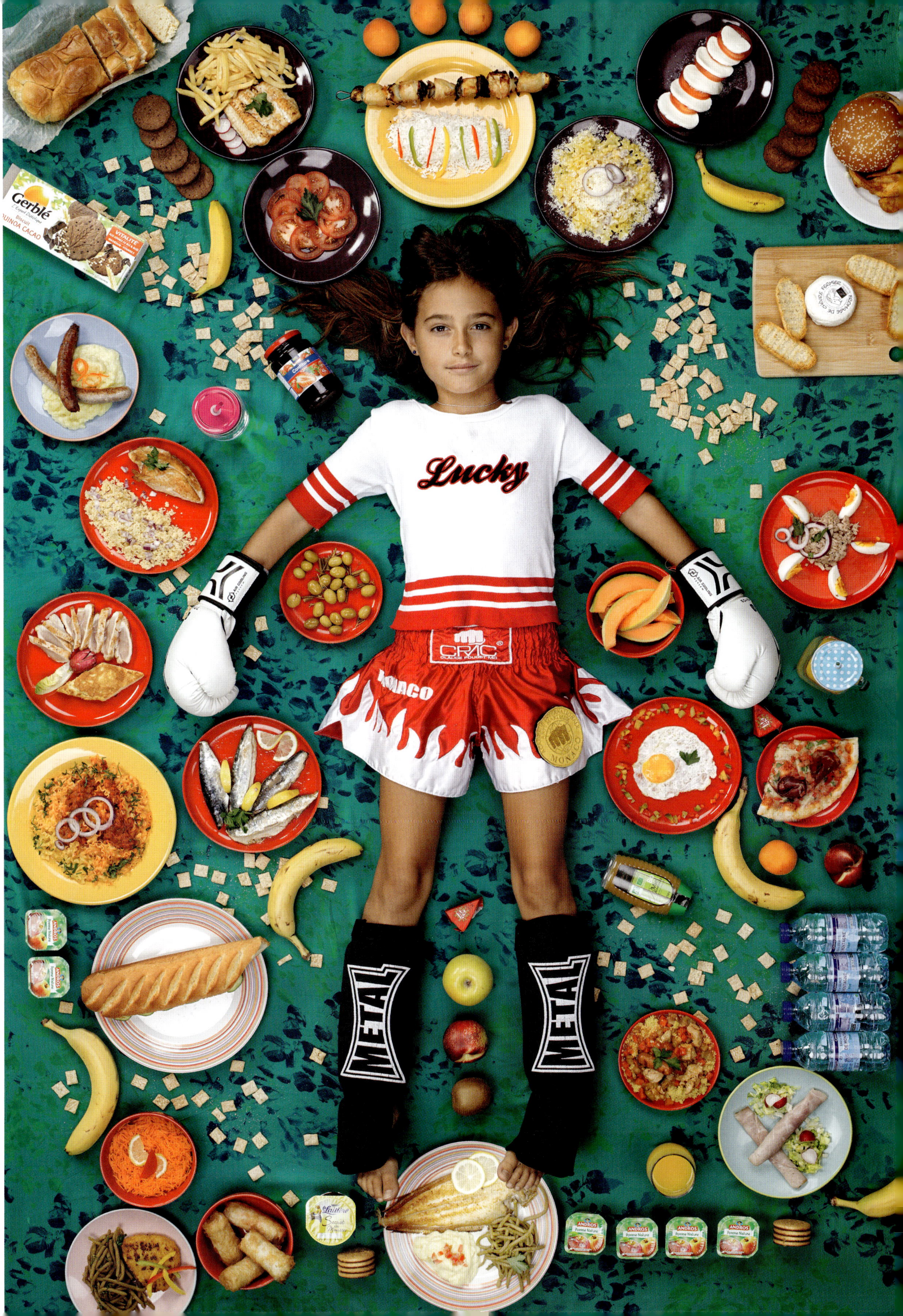
Gerblé
Lucky
CRAC
METAL
METAL

Isaiah Dedrick, 16

Long Beach, CA, USA.
Photographed March 20, 2016.

Isaiah was raised by his mother and grandmother, who does most of the cooking at home. One day, Isaiah would like to have enough space to grow his own garden. Isaiah's favorite food is orange chicken and fried rice and he loves the smell of apples sautéed with cinnamon. His mom doesn't permit him to drink soda and after this photo shoot, Isaiah decided to eliminate snacks from his diet. Isaiah's wish is that no one will go hungry in the world. He plays the drums and the flute and is studying acting. He'd like to be as funny as Eddie Murphy or Tyler Perry and be able to fly like Superman.

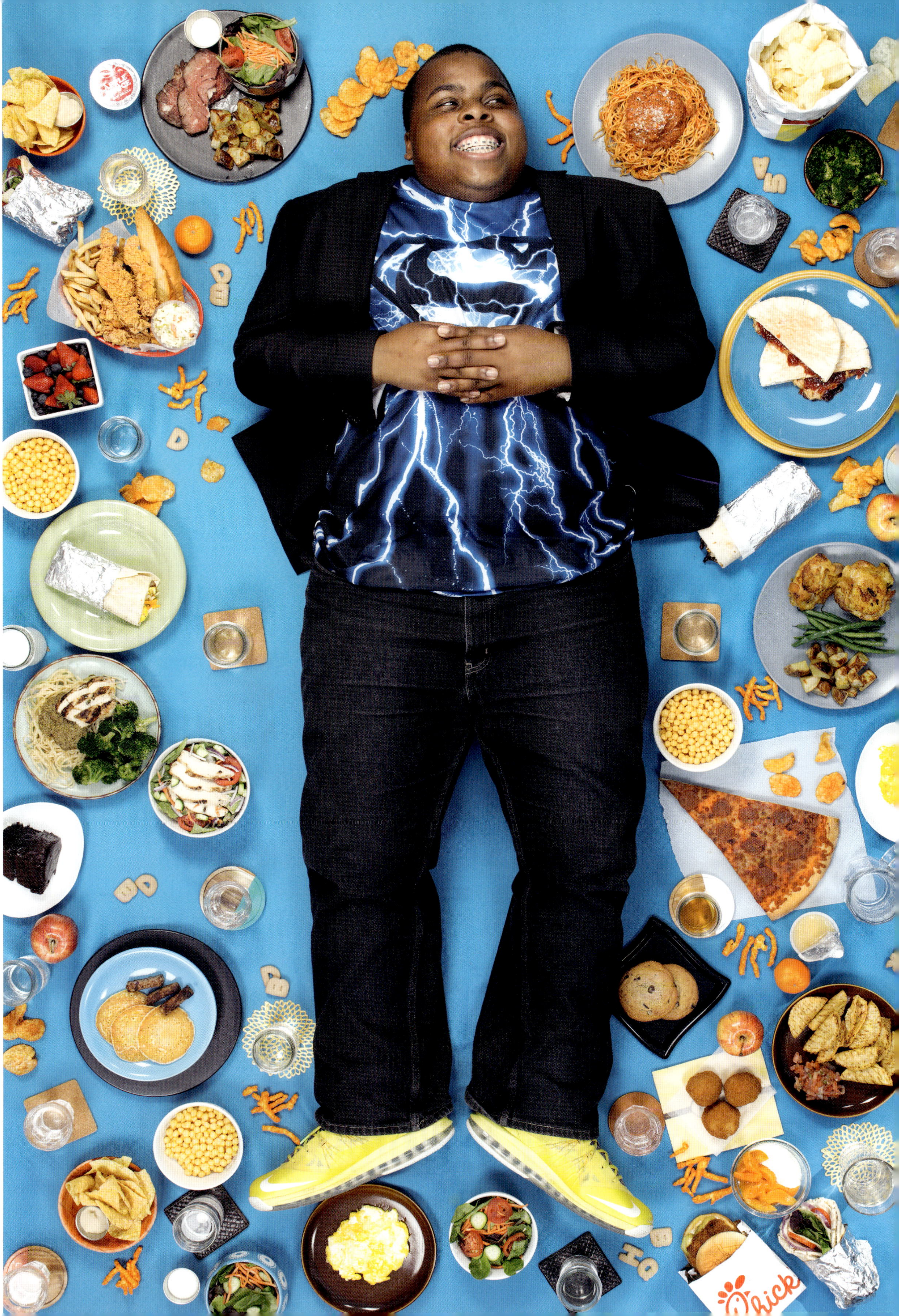

Daria Joy Cullen, 6

Los Angeles, California, USA.
Photographed February 21, 2016.

Daria loves bacon, pasta, popcorn slathered with butter, milk chocolate, and other sweets, particularly mint chocolate chip ice-cream. She won't eat fruits and vegetables of any kind, even as a toddler, not even mashed bananas or apple sauce. Her pediatrician is concerned about Daria's low weight and limited diet and her parents are concerned she may have an overactive gag reflex. Daria's role model is her big sister, who can make friends and play the violin effortlessly. For fun, Daria entertains her friends, impersonating a monkey. When she grows up, Daria would like to be a dog trainer. If she had enough money, she'd buy a horse and a pug.

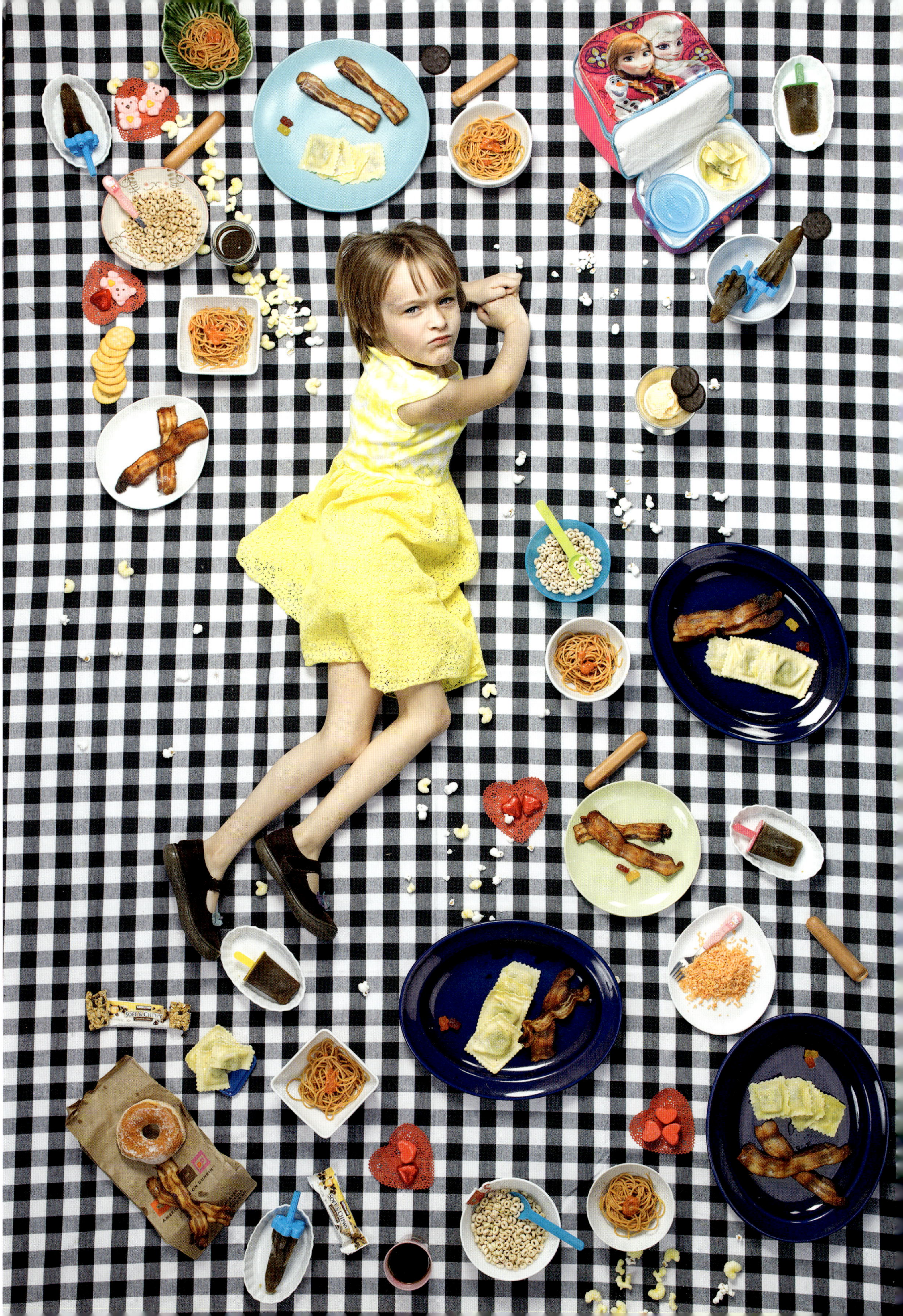

Majo Said, 7

Hamburg, Germany.
Photographed August 11, 2017.

Majo and his family fled Syria where his father had a small farm and his mother worked as a barber. Majo's favorite foods are dolmas with meatballs and ketchup. Until recently, he didn't care for pizza. At dinner, Majo always sits in the same place, second chair on the right. He and his family are Yazidis, a religion dating back to pre-Islamic times. Majo misses picking cherries and apples in Syria with his best friends Yusuf and Samed.

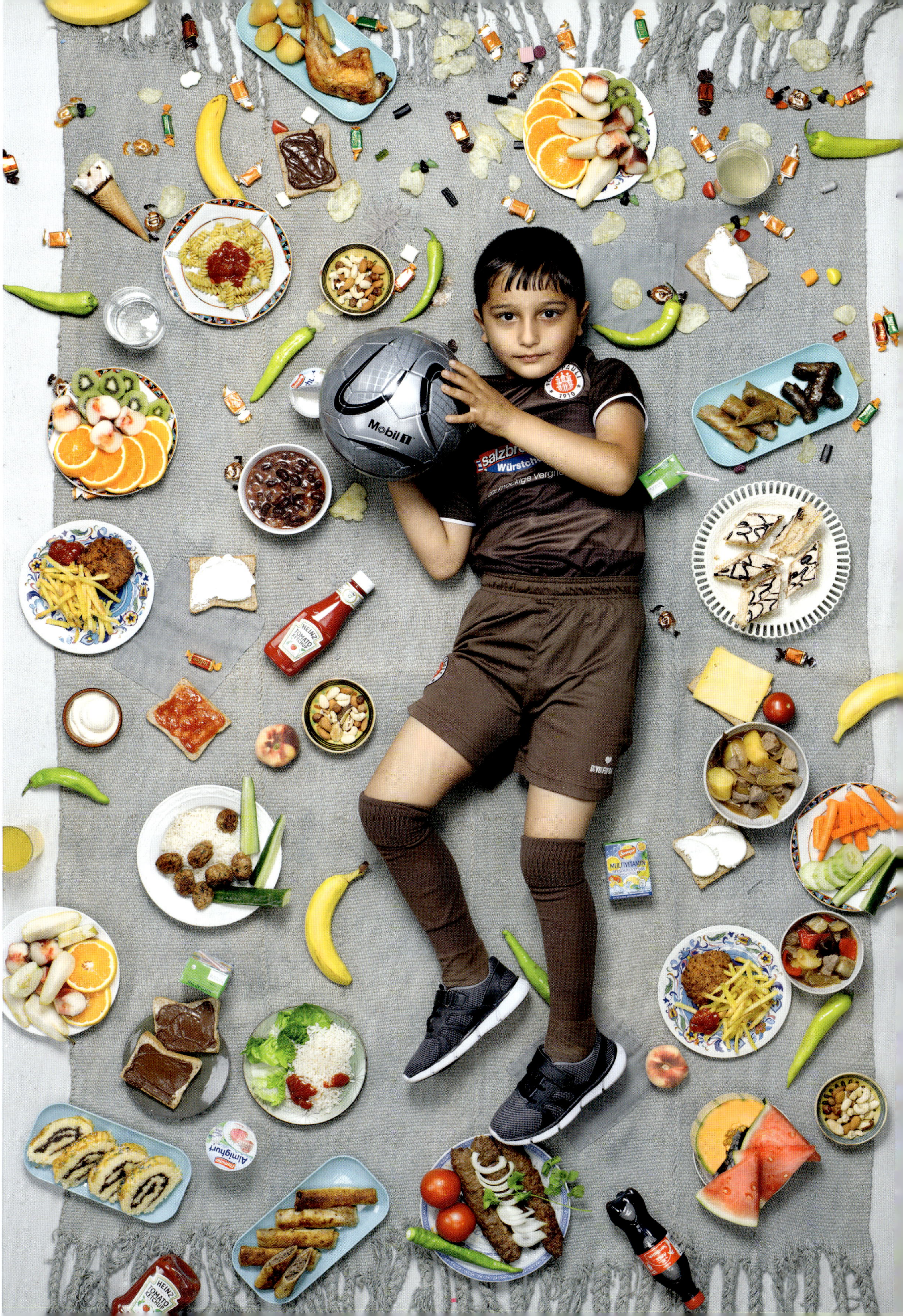
Mobil 1
HEINZ
TOMATO KETCHUP
MULTIVITAMIN
Almighurt

Wendy Cruz, 17

Los Angeles, CA, USA.
Photographed February 20, 2016.

Wendy lives with her parents and older sister in Koreatown, an ethnically diverse neighborhood near downtown Los Angeles where 2/3 of the residents were born outside the US. Wendy's dad is a cook in a Korean restaurant and sometimes mixes Korean and Central American food at home. Wendy remembers eating beef for the first time when she was about seven years old and not being able to stomach the taste. She passed the meat off to her sister who loved it. Later on, Wendy learned how animals were raised and slaughtered, reinforcing her commitment to being vegetarian.

After the photo shoot, Wendy saw how unhealthy she was (and how ironic it was that she was a vegetarian who didn't eat any vegetables). Growing up, it was hard being vegetarian in a home full of meat-eaters, so Wendy ate out a lot—at Denny's, Soup Plantation, and Buffalo Wild Wings (she'd have the mozzarella sticks or chips and dip). Since then though, Wendy eats more veggies and tries making dishes like zucchini casserole.

Wendy is intrigued by religious beliefs though she's an atheist. She discovered a book on Buddhism and has been guided by its lessons: don't stay mad at others and don't criticize, for instance. She tried meditation until her mom walked in on her and wondered what she was doing. Wendy likes shopping for clothes, too, especially shirts with unusual designs and graphics. She'd like to be a homicide detective, figuring out the how and why of murders. If she had the money, Wendy would buy a little house with a garden, just for herself.

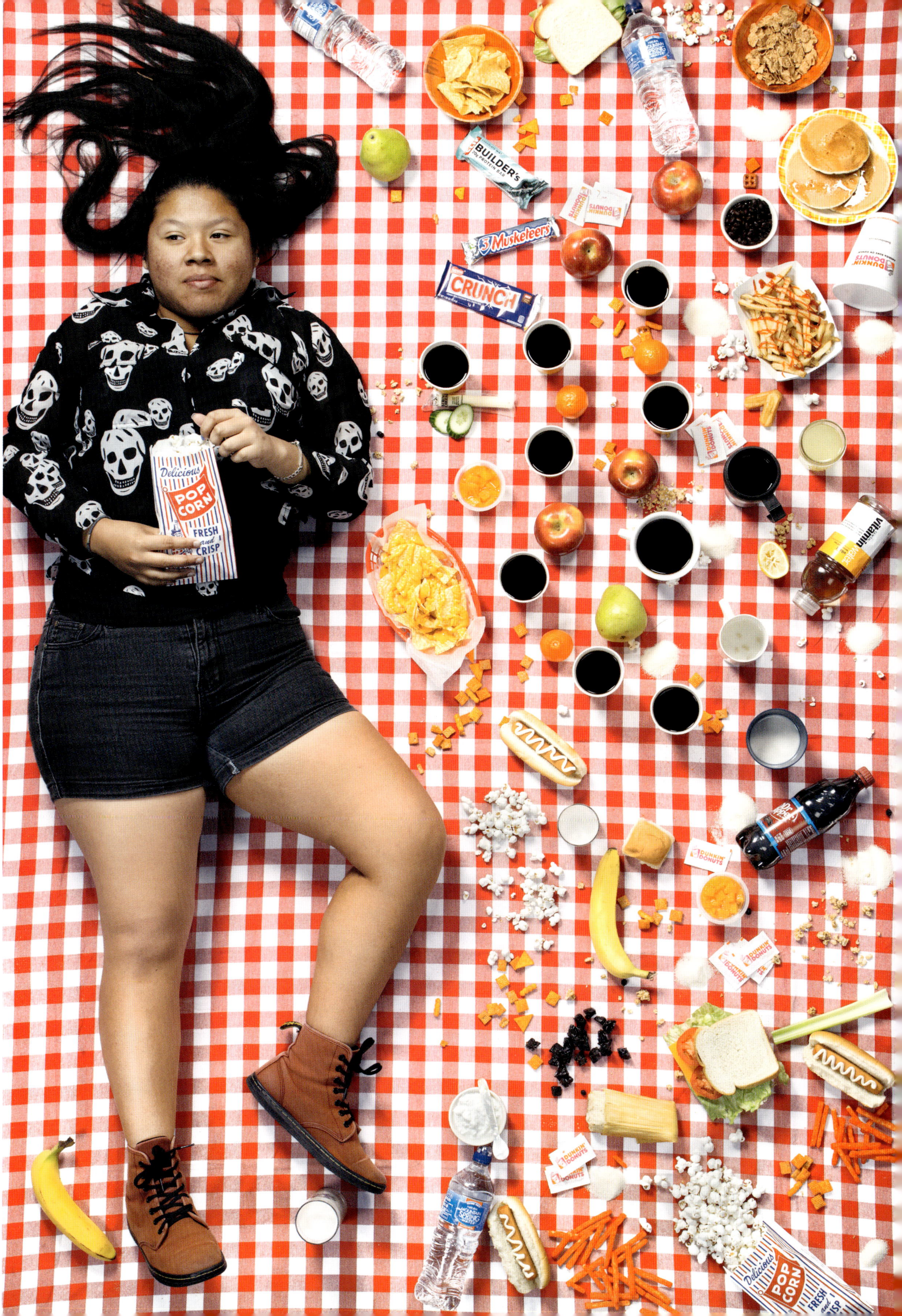
BUILDER's
3 Musketeers
CRUNCH
DUNKIN' DONUTS
Delicious
POP CORN
FRESH and CRISP
vitamin

Marek Strojvus, Jr., 7

New Haven, CT, USA.
Photographed December 8, 2017 in New York.

Marek, an only child, lives with his father, a single parent who makes his living as an electrical engineer, but who grew more focused on healthy eating once he became a father. He's since developed a social media following as a meal-prepper and crepe artist. Marek Jr. helps his dad prep their week's meals, cutting and seasoning vegetables, blending hummus, flipping oatmeal blueberry pancakes, shaping turkey meatballs, and parceling snacks. Marek's earliest memory of food is having an ice-cream cone with his "babka" at her village ice-cream parlor in Slovakia. When they visited her last summer, they helped harvest the fruits and vegetables in her garden and she rewarded them with bryndzové halušky, a classic, hearty Slovak meal made with dumplings and sheep's milk cheese sprinkled with bits of smoked pork fat. Marek's favorite foods are apples, strawberries with nut butter, crepes with chocolate, and creamy hummus. He's read all of the *Wimpy Kid Diaries*, treasures his Boston Bruins game puck and his Elf on the Shelf, and thinks sharks are cool. Marek's dream job is to be a marine and he'd like to drive a Bugatti Veyron, the world's most powerful car. When he falls asleep at night beside Squirtel (his blue, Pokémon turtle), Marek Jr. envisions scenes from favorite movies like *Sahara*.

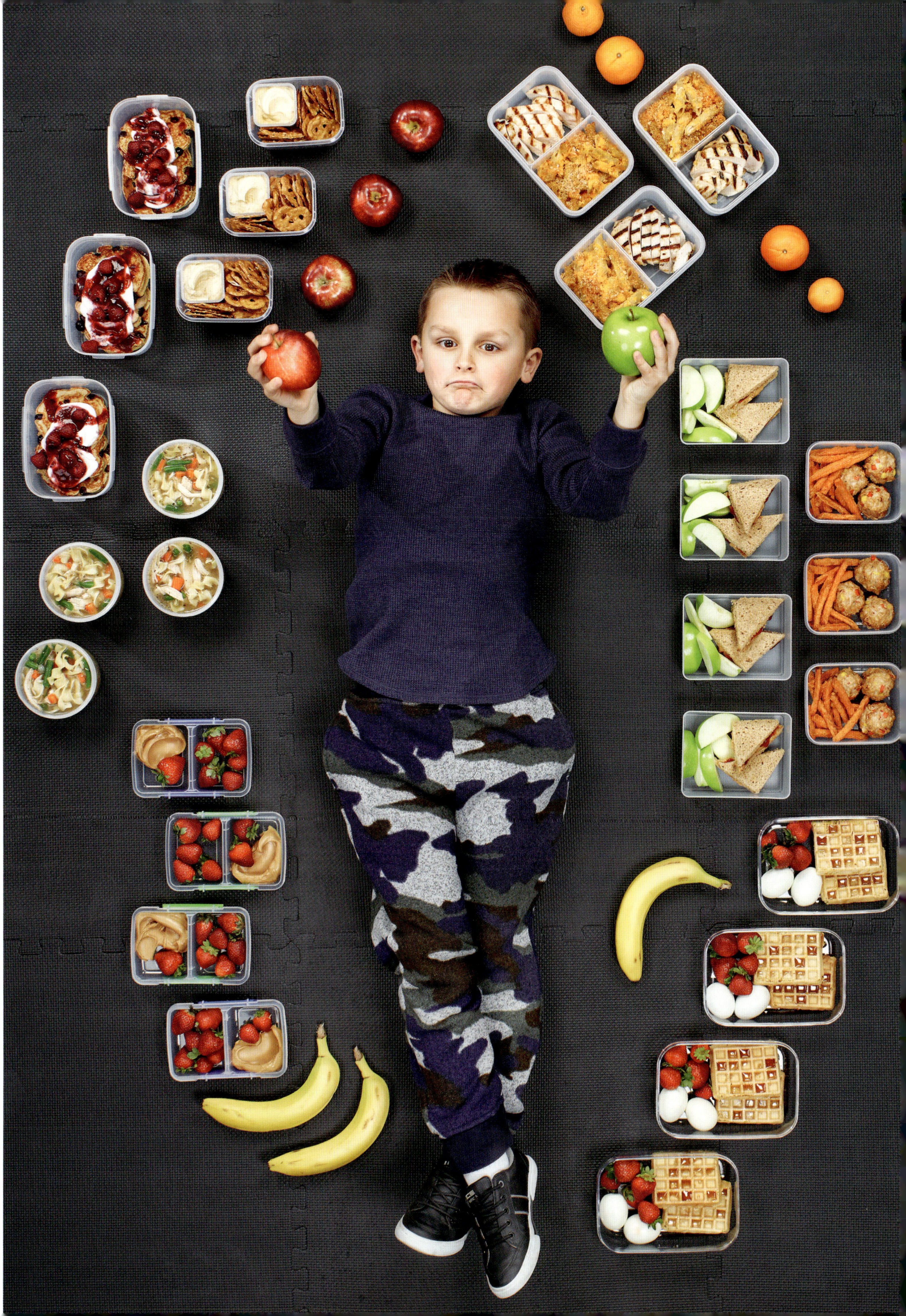

Anchal Sahani, 9

Chembur, India.
Photographed March 11, 2017.

Anchal lives in a tiny tin shack on a construction site in a suburb of Mumbai with her parents and two siblings. Her father makes less than $5 a day, just enough for her mother to prepare okra and cauliflower curry, lentils, and roti from scratch. Anchal would like to return to the farm where she was born in Bihar, go to school like other kids, and eventually become a teacher, but she's kept busy with household chores and looking after her baby brother. When she has time, she dresses up and leaves the construction site to enjoy the fragrance of jasmine and lotus and to watch the neighborhood kids playing cricket and running free. While on her walks, Anchal collects brightly colored chocolate wrappers she finds along the road. Anchal wishes her mother would love her the way she loves her baby brother.

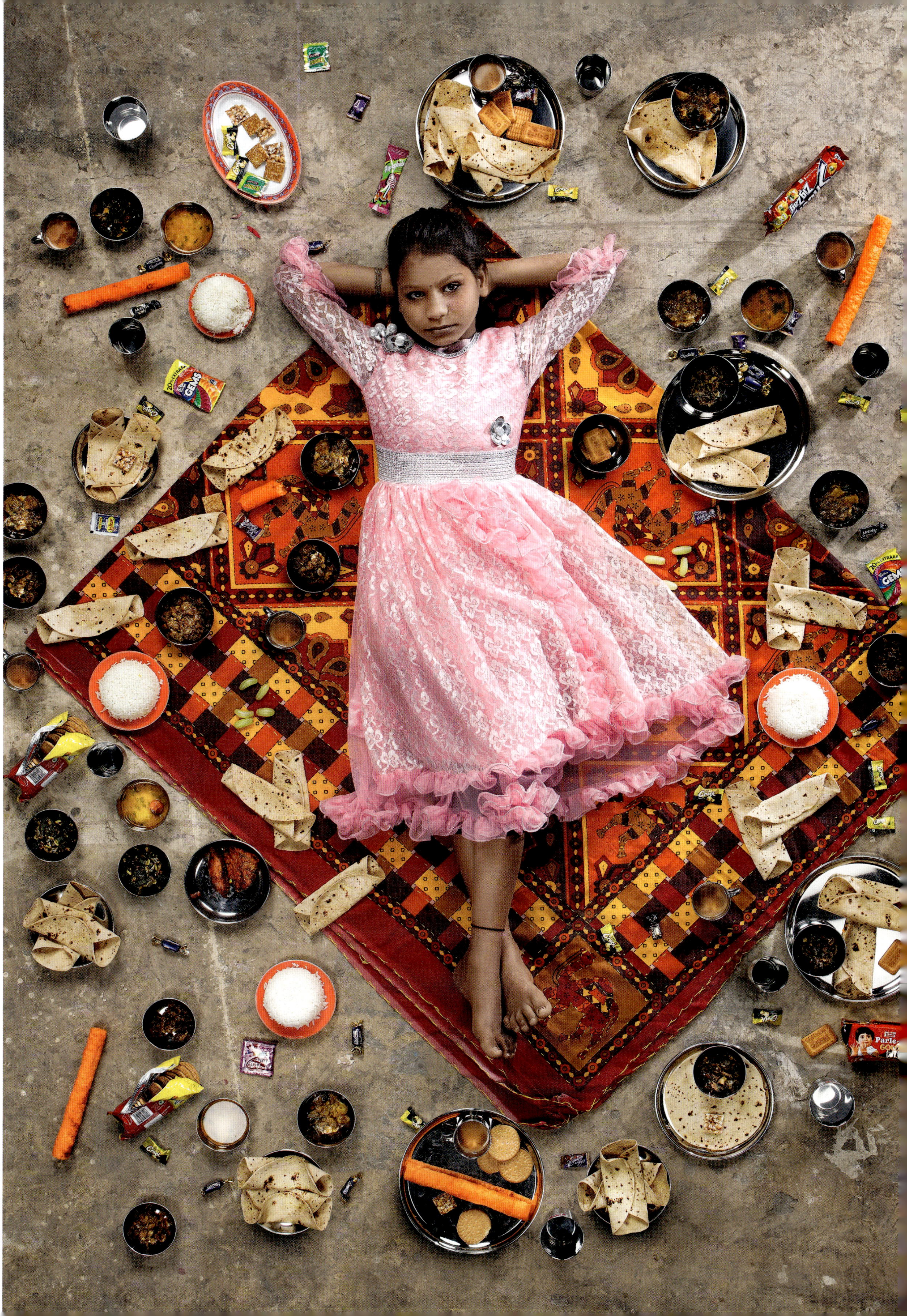
GEMS

Saifullah Bin Sohail, 12

Dubai, UAE.
Photographed August 12, 2018.

Saifullah lives in an apartment with his parents and four siblings. His father is a used car salesman and his mother teaches Islamic studies. Saifullah has a talent for making animal noises—cats, dogs, sheep, pigs, and cows—and this is how he gets people to laugh. Saifullah dreams of becoming a successful aeronautical engineer, designing commercial jets, and one day buying a great big house where he'll live with his parents. When he goes to sleep at night, Saifullah thinks of food, and pizza in particular. Saifullah's earliest memory of food was his first taste of biriyani in Pakistan where his grandparents still live. They were once farmers, growing mangoes and dates and their diet was better than his. They never ate pizza.

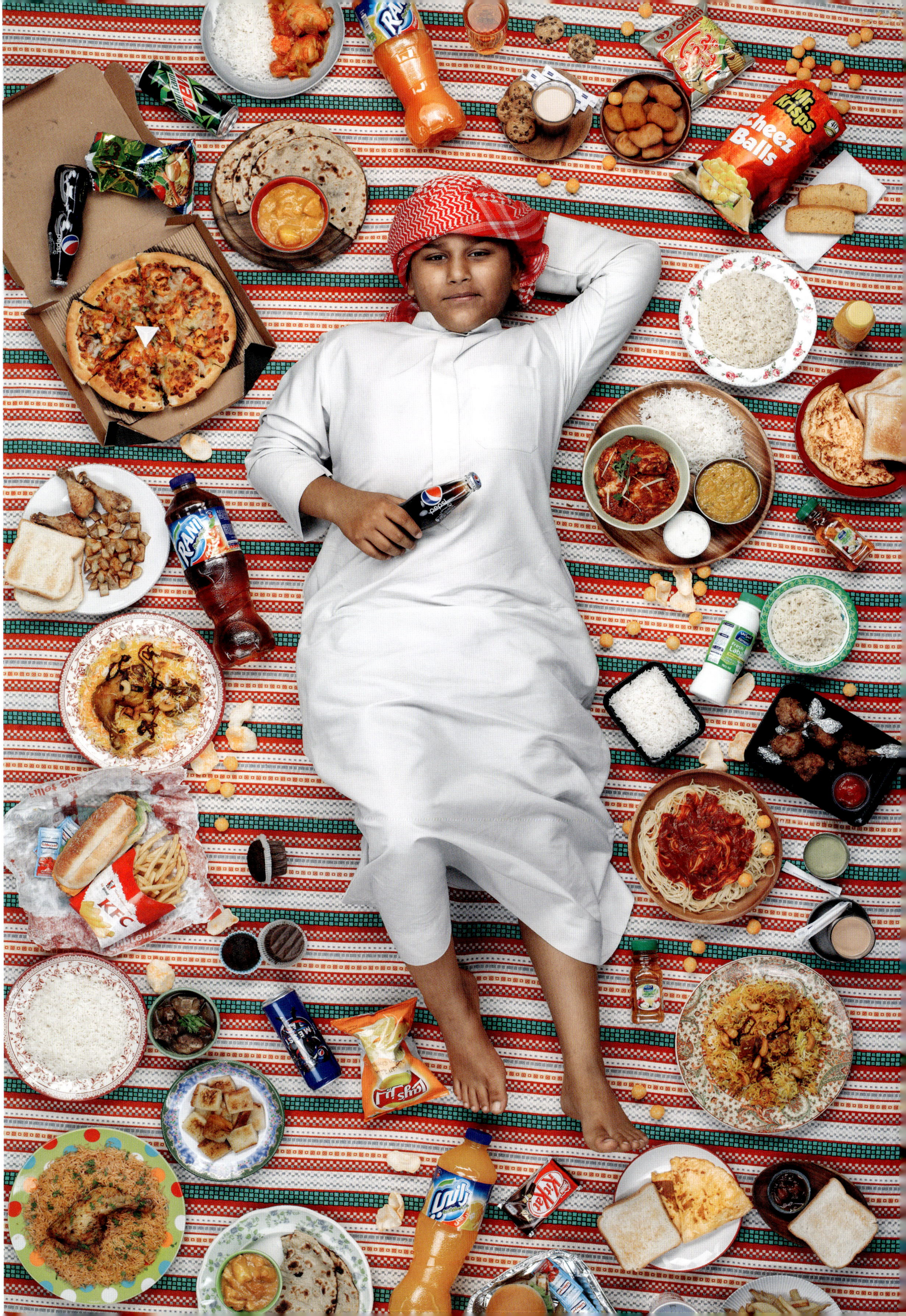
Mr. Krisps
Cheez Balls
KFC

Ayme Boquadi, 7

Brasilia, Brazil.
Photographed August 19, 2018.

Ayme, an only child, has been raised on a mostly indigenous diet. Her dad is a forest engineer and nutritionist and her mom researches the culinary and medicinal uses of foods from the Cerrado region of Brazil. Ayme's mother prepares dishes like walnut cassava moqueca and cauliflower soufflé with cupuaçu cream at her restaurant, Buriti Zen. Ayme's earliest memory of food is her mama's milk. Thinking of this makes her want to return to that time and nurse again. Açai is Ayme's favorite food and part of her heritage; her great-grandmother was an açai merchant who sold her berries at Ver-o-peso Market in Belém. Ayme has helped her mom grow and harvest many fruits and vegetables: acerola, blackberry, pitanga (a Brazilian cherry), lemons, mexerica (tangerine), cabbage, basil, and lettuce. From participating in Daily Bread, Ayme learned that she eats many things that other children don't eat—like lots of fresh vegetables.

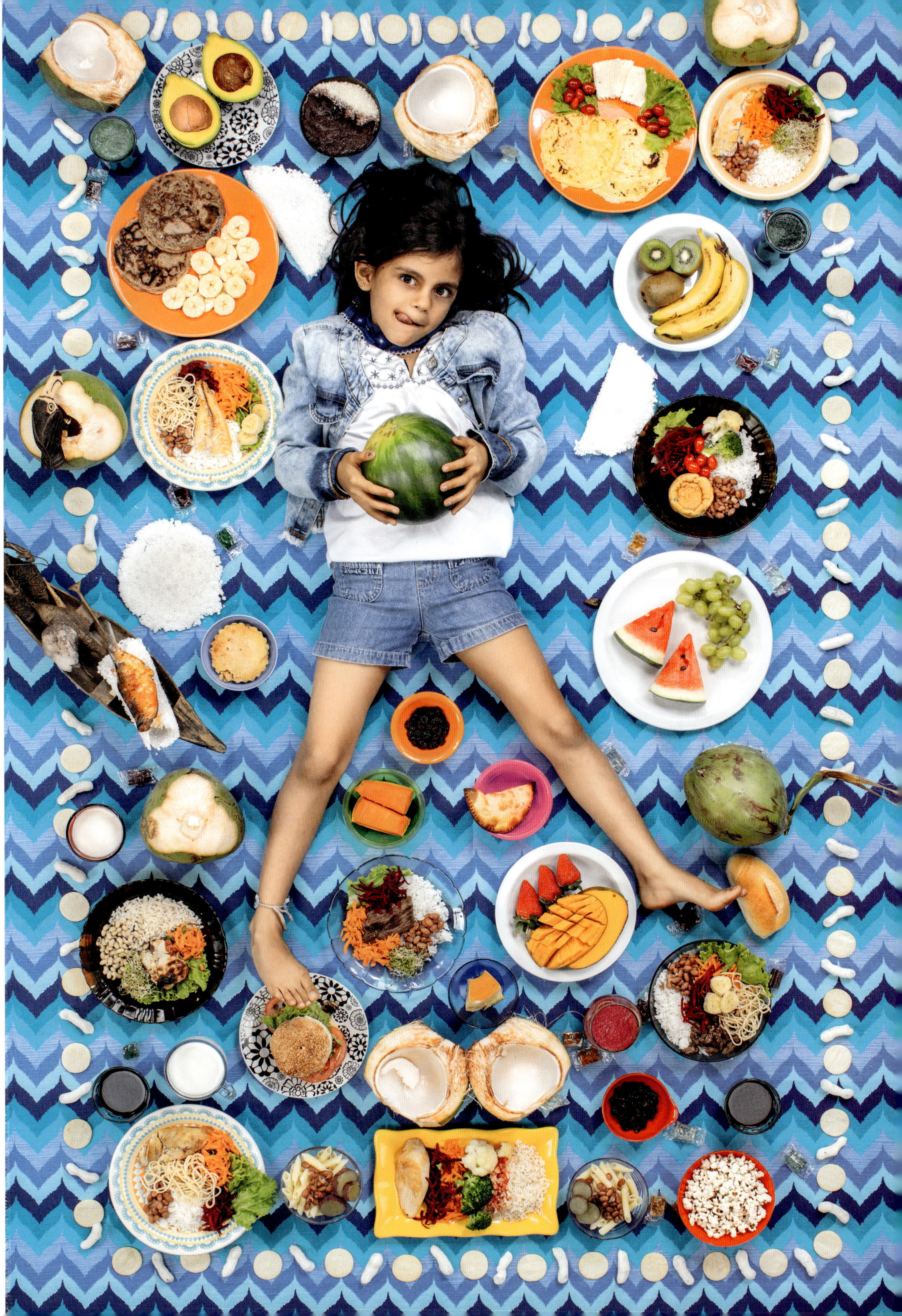

Bradley Choi, 9

Temple City, CA, USA.
Photographed March 20, 2016.

Bradley, a boy of few words, lives in the San Gabriel Valley, northeast of Los Angeles, with his parents and younger brother. Bradley's favorite food is sushi. He dislikes shrimp and mushrooms and observed that he doesn't eat enough greens. He loves to read and swim and enjoys helping others. Before going to sleep, Bradley prays that he will do well in school. He also wishes his parents would let him have a small, fluffy dog. When he grows up, Bradley wants to be a dentist.

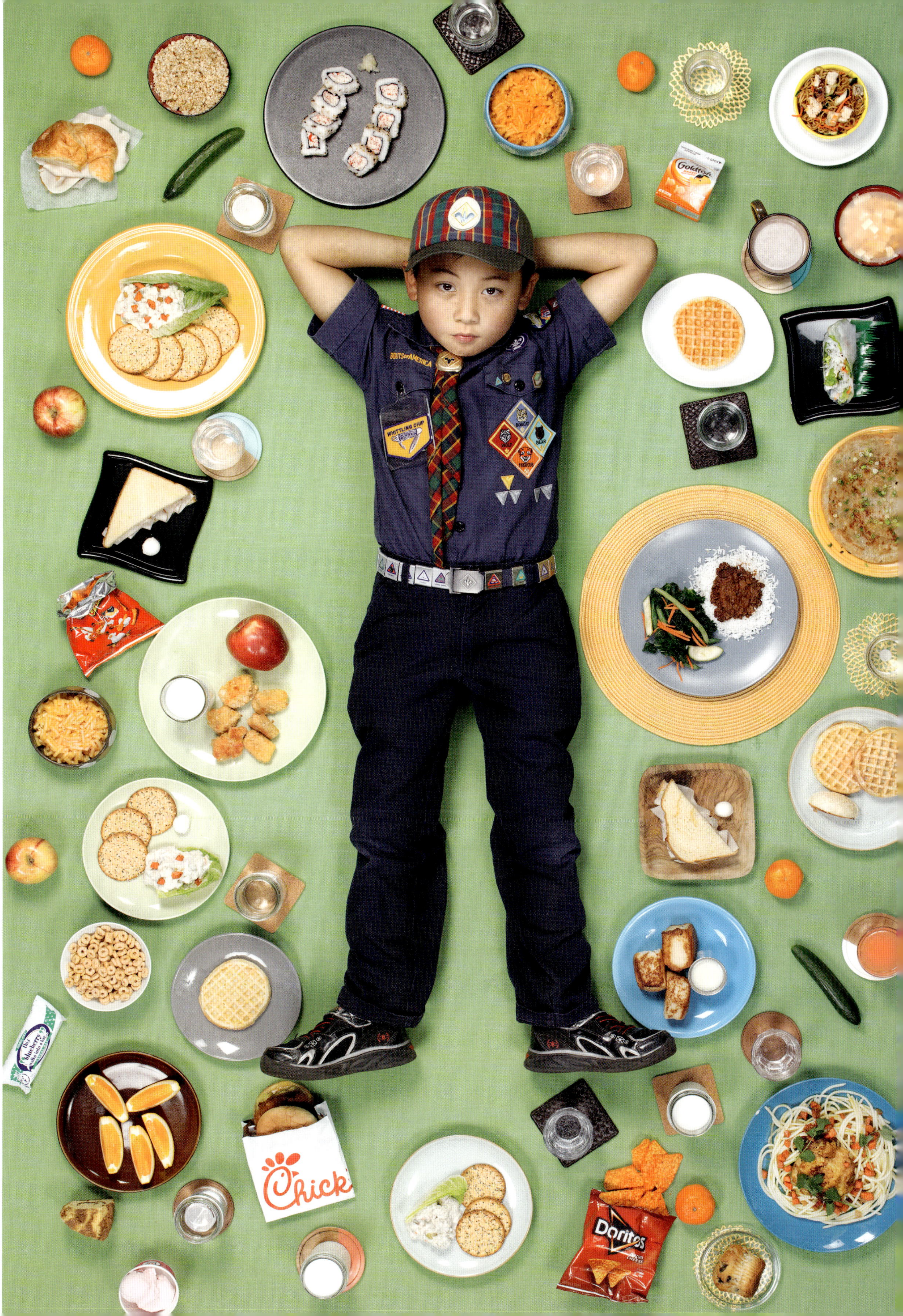
Goldfish
WHITTLING CHIP
Chick
Doritos

Carolina Bonet Sanabrais, 5

Los Angeles, CA, USA.
Photographed January 30, 2016.

Carolina is being raised by her two moms. One is a clinical oncology social worker, the other is an art historian and does most of the cooking. Carolina's favorite food is turron, a Filipino desert made with jackfruit and banana. Carolina has grown tomatoes, cilantro, and has a lime tree in her yard. She collects dead beetles, butterflies, flowers, shells, and rocks. She's taking diving classes at UCLA and teaches other kids to do cartwheels. She would like to be a vet when she grows up.

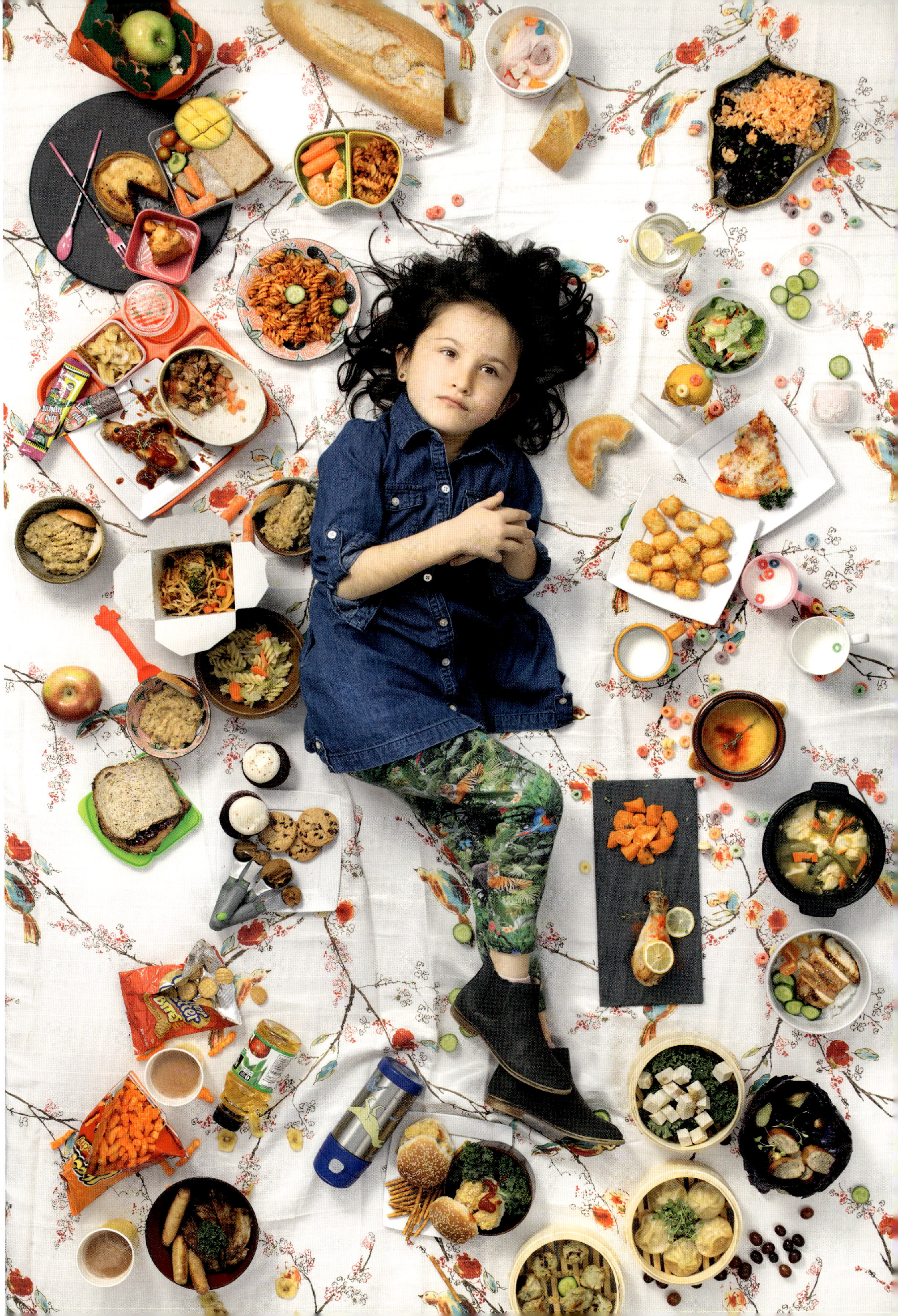

Sira Cissokho, 11

Tambacounda, Senegal.
Photographed August 30, 2017 in Dakar.

Sira, one of nine children, is from Tambacounda, about seven hours north of Dakar. Sira's father is a musician and her mother is a housewife. Sira doesn't always get enough to eat. On special occasions, Sira's mom makes her favorite dish, chicken. Many of the foods Sira and her family eat are grown in their garden, including millet and peanuts. Sira has learned to cook ngalakh, a Senegalese millet porridge. If she had enough money, Sira would buy her parents a trip to Mecca. Of all her possessions, the thing Sira cherishes most is a bracelet her grandfather passed down to her before he died.

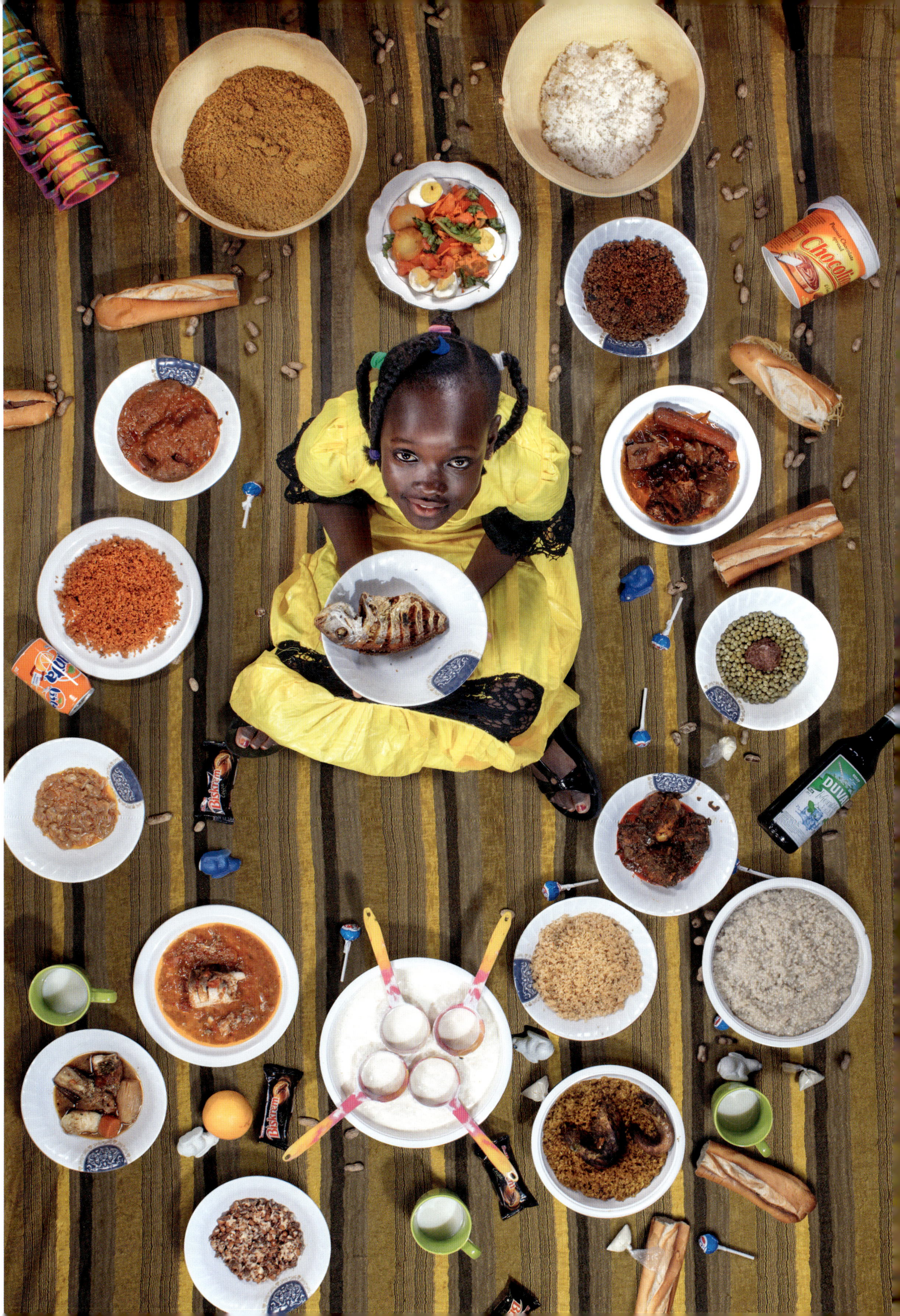
Biskrem

Paolo Mendolaro, 9

Belpasso, Sicily, Italy.
Photographed August 23, 2017 in Catania.

Paolo and his family of four live in an apartment in Belpasso, a tiny medieval village on the east coast of Sicily, founded in 1305. When he steps outside his apartment, Paolo sees the center square and Mother Church of Belpasso with its lava-stone staircase and bell tower. Paolo's mom works full time for a cosmetics company, but makes time to prepare homemade meals for her family like Sicilian cannoli and pasta alla Norma. Once a week, they buy a roast chicken or go out for pizza, which Paolo loves most of all. Paolo has learned to make his own pizza and pasta as well as biscuits and big donuts. His grandfather had an overflowing garden and Paolo helped harvest eggplants, zucchini, bell peppers, olives, strawberries, peaches, tomatoes, peas, and fava beans. During the week that Paolo kept his journal for Daily Bread, he'd been going to the beach with his family and didn't follow as healthy a diet as usual; they often ate fast food. Paolo keeps his parents in his prayers. For his mother, he wishes for a dryer machine, and a new truck for his father, a carpenter. If he had enough money, Paolo would buy a PlayStation 4, a giant Lego set and, at minimum, a one-week holiday for the whole family.

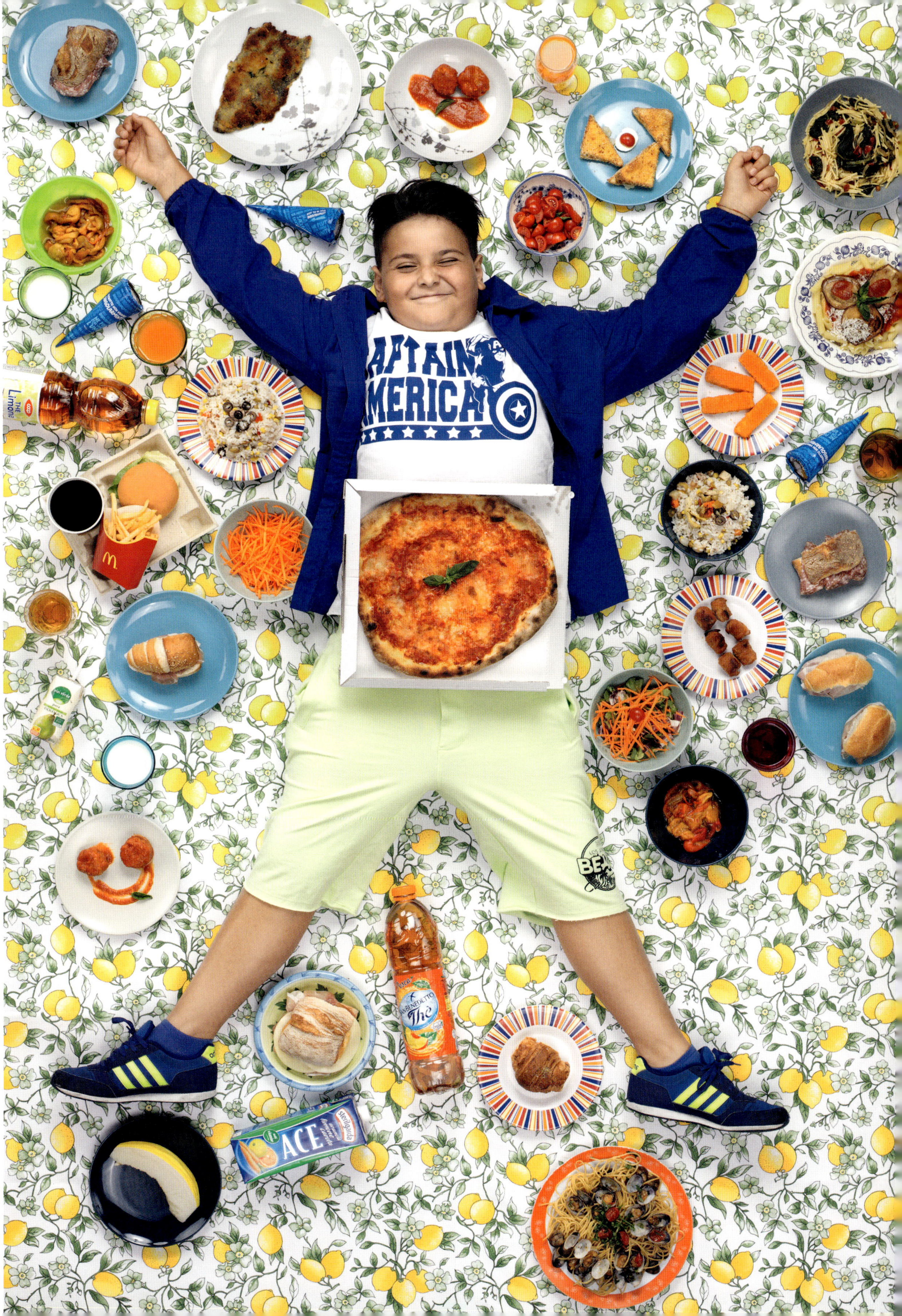

APTAIN
MERICA
ACE

Ademilson Francisco dos Santos, 11

Vão de Almas, Goiás, Brazil.
Photographed August 19, 2018 in Brasilia.

Ademilson is from Vão de Almas, a community of 300 families in the Cerrado region of Goiás. Ademilson's home is 200 kilometers from the nearest town, a journey on mountainous, unpaved roads through valleys and across rivers—an almost impossible trip during the rainy season. There is no TV, electricity, or running water. Villagers bathe, wash their clothes, and clean their pots and pans in the Capivara River. Ademilson, the youngest of seven children, goes to school in the morning (an hour's walk from home) and in the afternoon returns to help his father with farming and collecting native plants. The family cultivates a cornucopia of crops: rice, manihot (cassava), sweet potatoes, squash, beans, gherkin, okra, jiló, orange, lemon, watermelon, corn, coffee, and sugar cane. They collect a bounty of native fruits, too: buriti, mangaba, mango, jatobá, pequi, caju, and coco indaiá. They produce coconut oil, mamona oil (castor oil), and sesame and peanut paçoca (similar to peanut brittle). They farm without the use of machinery, irrigation, or pesticides and fertilize with ash from the burning of the bush. Manihot, the brown root in the upper right-hand corner of the photograph, is a staple of Ademilson's diet. His favorite treats are mangoes and paçoca. There are many kinds of food Ademilson doesn't eat because they're not part of his diet and are completely foreign. He tried a hot dog when he went to the city and hated it. He'd never eaten pizza before coming to Braslila to be photographed. In his portrait, Ademilson is holding buriti, a wild palm from the Cerrado rich in carotenoids and antioxidants which indigenous people refer to as the "tree of life" because of its many uses: its wood goes into the construction of homes and handcrafts; leaves are used to cover houses; fibers are used to make textiles; and the orange pulp of the fruit is used for food. Even the seeds of the buriti fruit aren't wasted—they're cold pressed by natives who use the oil to protect themselves from the sun and soothe sore muscles.

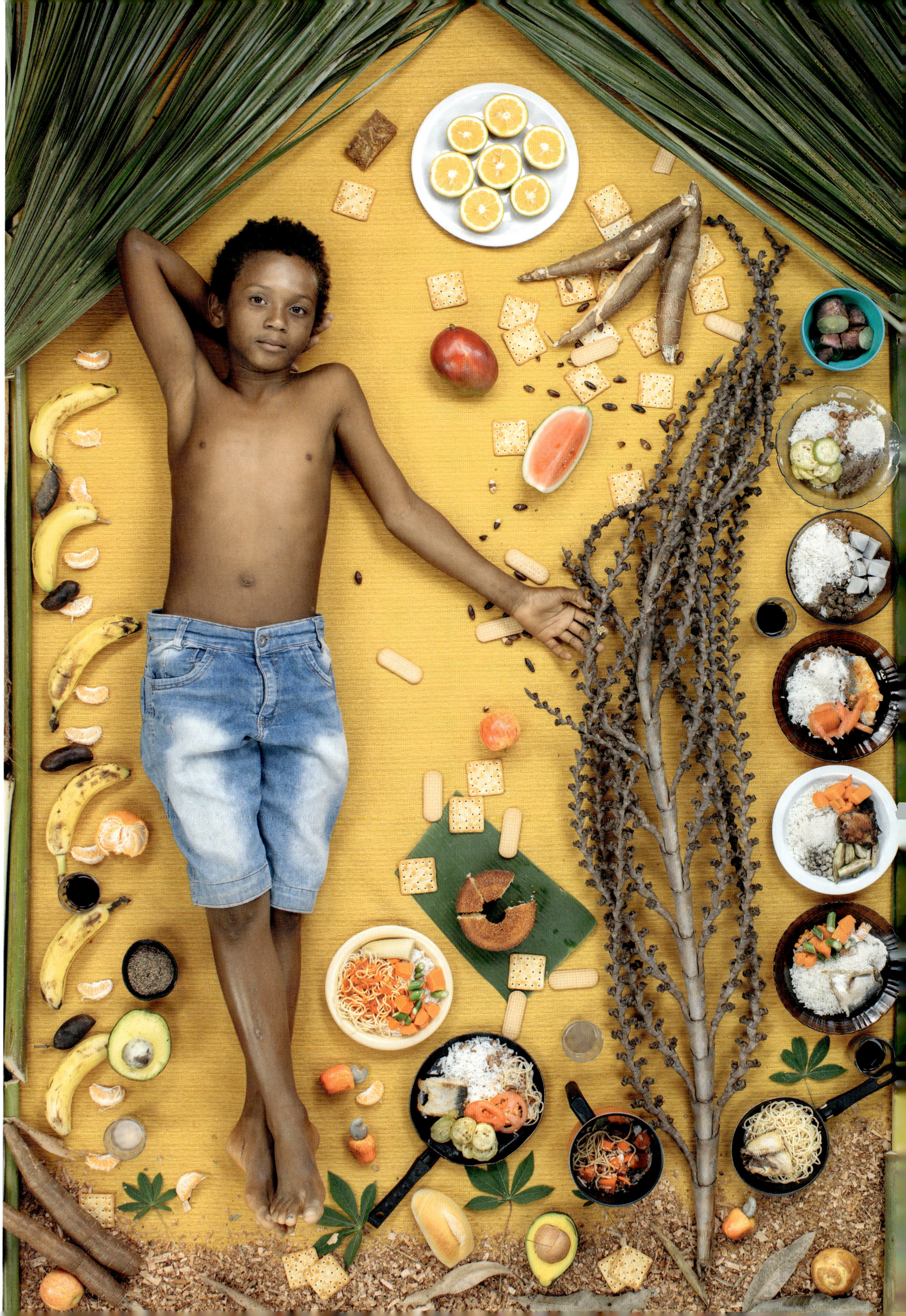

Nino Khaburzania, 6

West Hollywood, CA, USA.
Photographed March 19, 2016.

Nino lives in a West Hollywood apartment surrounded by tall palms with her littler sister, her mom, an ultrasound technician, and dad, a chess player. Nino's diet is a mix of traditional Georgian dishes (her Grandma Tisiana's specialties) and American staples: khachapuri (cheese filled bread), gomi (cornmeal with sulguni cheese), mchadi (cornbread), pizza, bean and cheese nachos, and cheese quesadillas. She's also fond of Chinese chow mein noodles and orange chicken at Panda Express, Happy Meals from McDonald's, Double Doubles from In-N-Out Burger, sandwiches from Subway, pancakes from IHOP, chocolate frappuccinos from Starbucks, and just about anything from The Cheesecake Factory. Nino's hobbies include collecting L.O.L. Surprise dolls, drawing, and singing and dancing like Jojo Siwa, her favorite YouTube personality. Nino would like to be a very famous actress and a very famous person. If she had the money, she would buy books and toys for needy kids.

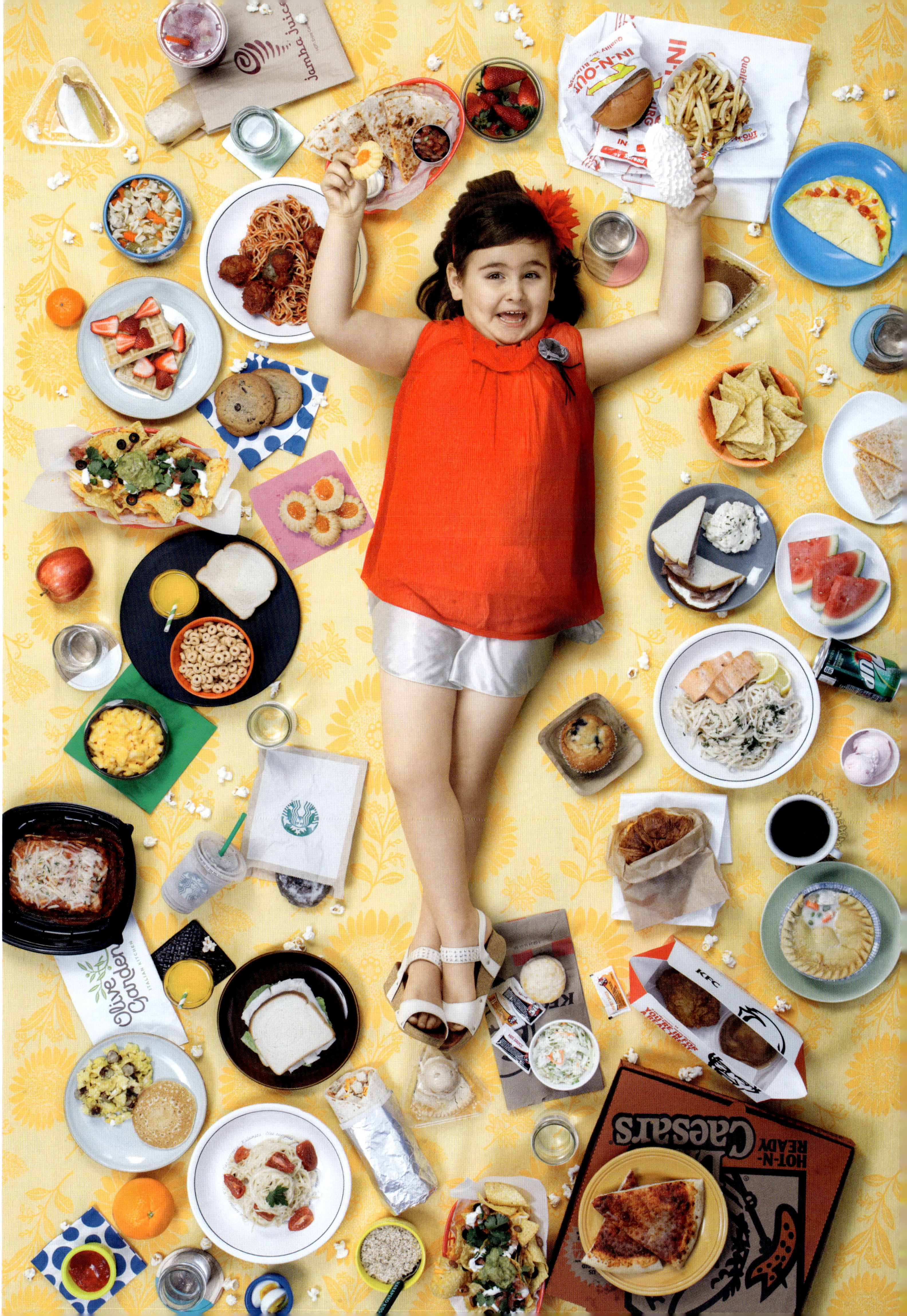
Jamba Juice
IN-N-OUT
Olive Garden
ITALIAN KITCHEN
KFC
HOT-N-READY
Caesars
7up

Frank Fadel Agbomenou, 8

Dakar, Senegal.
Photographed August 30, 2017.

Frank lives with his older brother and father, a human resources manager, in an apartment in a posh neighborhood of Dakar. Frank would like to see his dad and mum together again but he doesn't think that wish will be fulfilled. Frank cried a couple weeks ago; his mum told him she would take him to the beach but then changed her mind. She's busy, working as a caterer for parties and fancy hotel events. There is almost nothing Frank doesn't like to eat. He eats lots of peanuts from the peanut tree on his terrace. He's especially fond of fish and the family cook knows how to prepare it just right. Frank is an excellent dancer and has mastered summersaults though he prefers watching TV and playing games on his PlayStation. The thing that makes him laugh the hardest is when his cousin Coco falls down. Frank dreams of buying a flashy sports car and traveling to Paris. When he grows up, he wants to be a gynecologist.

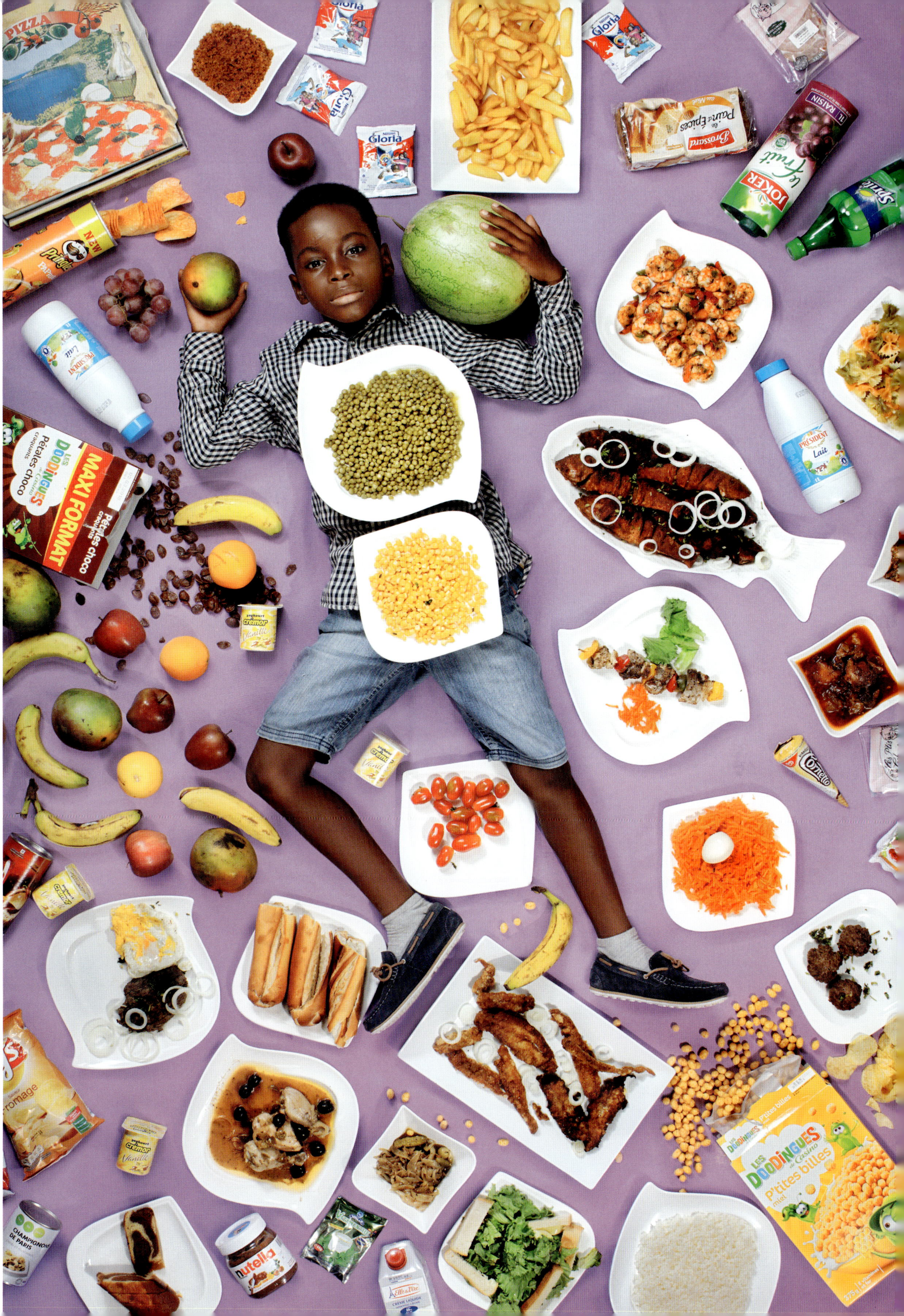

PIZZA
Gloria
MAXI FORMAT
Pétales choco
LES DOODINGUES
Pain d'Épices
Brossard
JOKER
le fruit
RAISIN
Sprite
PRÉSIDENT
Lait
cremor
Vanille
Cornetto
P'tites billes
nutella
CHAMPIGNONS DE PARIS

Praneeta Karandikar, 10

Mumbai, India.
Photographed March 12, 2017.

Praneeta's family of six live in a tiny one-room house (10 x 15 feet) in Govandi, a congested suburban neighborhood of Mumbai. When she steps out of her house, Praneeta sees busy, narrow lanes, water storage tanks, and a small corner where she grows potted plants. Her mother, the bread-winner of the family, is a fish monger, which is why there's so much fish in Praneeta's diet. She loves sour food most, though hot and spicy dishes are among her favorites, too, like pav bhaji which is made from fresh vegetables mashed and cooked together in a thick, spicy curry and served with bread fried in butter. Praneeta's earliest memory of food is strawberry-flavored falooda, a desert made with vermicelli, rose syrup, sweet basil seeds, milk, and ice-cream. Praneeta's parents take turns cooking meals at home—dad covers lunch and mom dinner after she comes home from work late in the evening. They seldom eat out. Once in a while, she'll have a McDonald's burger, but it's very expensive and not as healthy as the food they eat at home. Praneeta loves acting and dancing and even received awards from her school for her one-act play in Marathi. She's good at karate and badminton and has taught herself to swim by jumping into the deep well in her village. She wants to be a great choreographer when she grows up, inspired by Madhuri Dixit, a Bollywood actress and dancer. If she had the money, Praneeta would spend it on getting her mother's knees replaced at a good hospital. She wishes her mother didn't have to work so hard and that her father could find work and spend less time drinking.

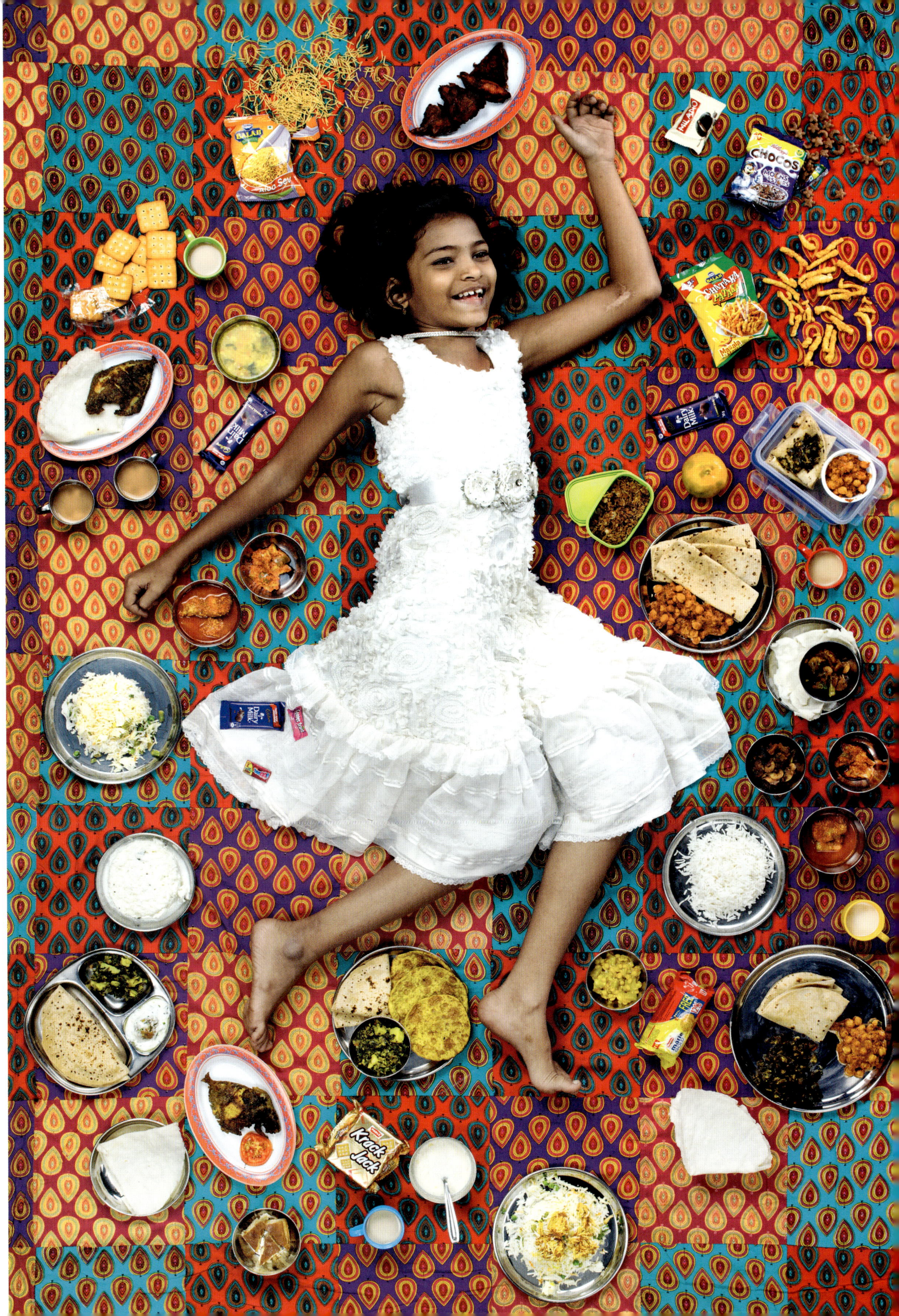
BALAJI
Aloo Sev
CHOCOS
Dairy Milk
Krack Jack

Soulaymane Landim Silva Fernandes, 8

Nice, France.
Photographed August 18, 2017.

Soulay's grandparents came to France from Morroco and his grandpa supported the family, working as a crane operator. Soulay's family is Muslim and celebrates the end of Ramadan with the sacrifice of a sheep, which they serve with couscous and many little cakes. The healthiest food Soulay eats is the fish and vegetables his mother makes. The unhealthiest is the fish he gets from McDonald's (no more than three times a month). Soulay's father wakes at 4:00 a.m. to deliver wholesale fruits and vegetables to restaurants all over Nice. His mom works in the surgical department of a hospital, preparing patients for their operations. Soulay often sees his mother helping other people like the Bosnian mom with nine children who lives in the street year round. They give her clothes, food, and sometimes money. Soulay admires his mom's generosity. She fights against food waste, collecting unsold food and distributing it where there is need. She knows many things and is beautiful. She takes Soulay and his sister everywhere, too—the playground, the circus, the cinema. The only thing missing in Soulay's life is his big uncle Mohamed who died of lung cancer in Morocco because he didn't have money to be cured in a hospital. He had a little fruit and vegetable shop and if somebody poor came in, he gave them food without asking for money. Soulay would like to be a judoka (professional judo trainer) and to be invisible to make people laugh or frighten them. Sometimes, Soulay has nightmares of thieves who catch hold of him, but when he wakes, he is safe in his room surrounded by his books, his posters of Fortnite and the Nice futbol team, and his favorite toy, Capitaine Crochet.

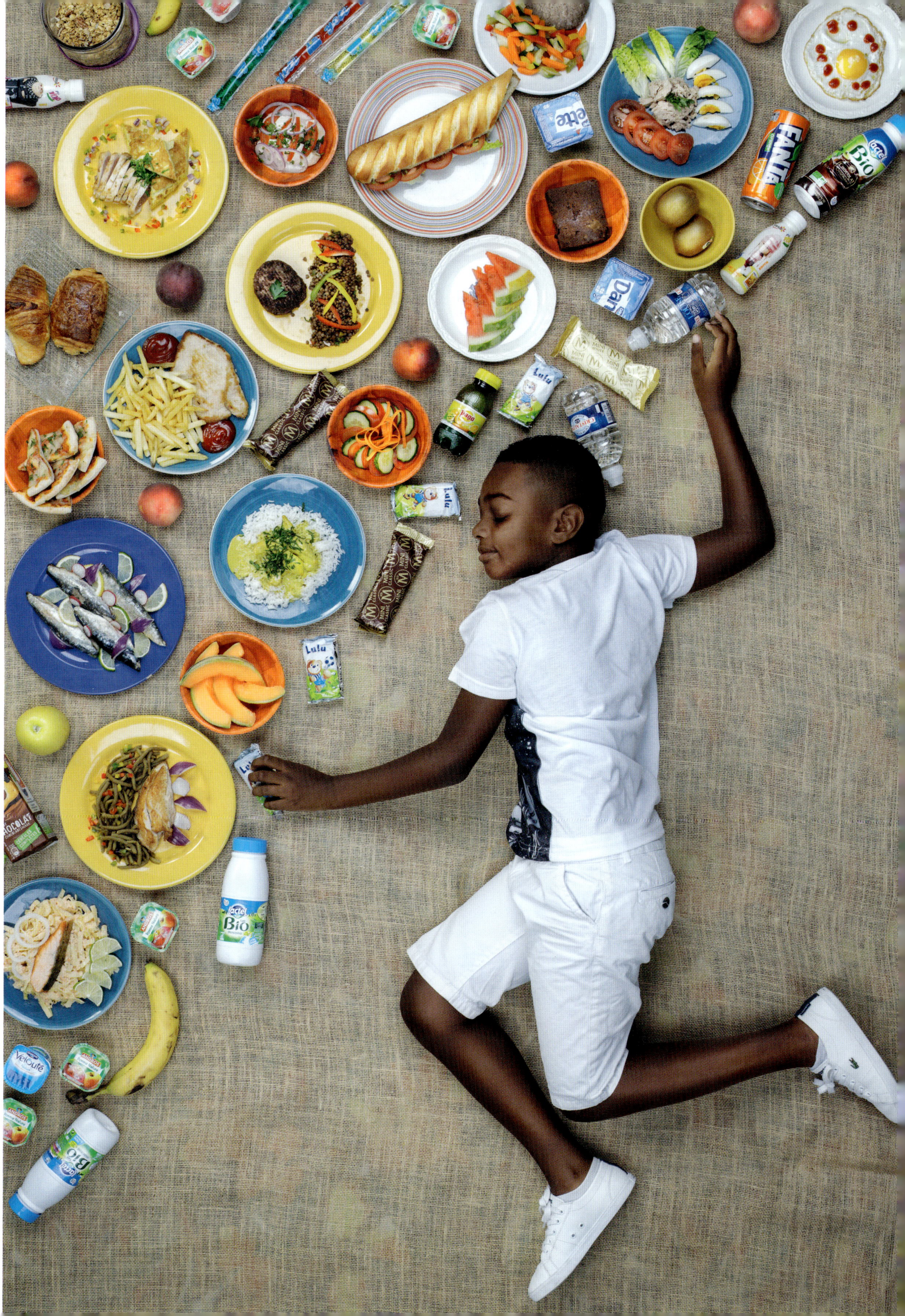
FANTA
Bio
Lulu
Velouté

Hank Segal, 8

Altadena, CA, USA.
Photographed January 30, 2016.

Hank lives with his mom, a voice teacher, his father, a photographer, and their dog, Django near the foothills of the San Gabriel Mountains northeast of Los Angeles. Hank and his parents have grown sun gold cherry tomatoes, artichokes, zucchini, spinach, pomegranates, yams, snap peas, watercress, rosemary, thyme, basil, serrano chili peppers, boysenberries, Kyoho grapes, raspberries, rhubarb, and watermelon. Hank has an adventurous palette. While eating a fried branzino at a Lebanese restaurant, he announced, "I'm gonna' get all Anthony Bourdain on it!" and popped the fish's crispy eyeball in his mouth. Usually, Hank and his parents talk politics over dinner or succumb to TV. Hank likes his back scratched and figures he must be part dog because his sense of smell is so keen. He especially likes the aroma of melted butter and garlic. He also likes 80s music because "they really knew how to use the synth." Hank's heroes are Albert Einstein, Teddy Roosevelt, and Abe Lincoln because he fixed slavery and has a sweet beard. Hank wants to be a mechanical engineer at NASA when he grows up.

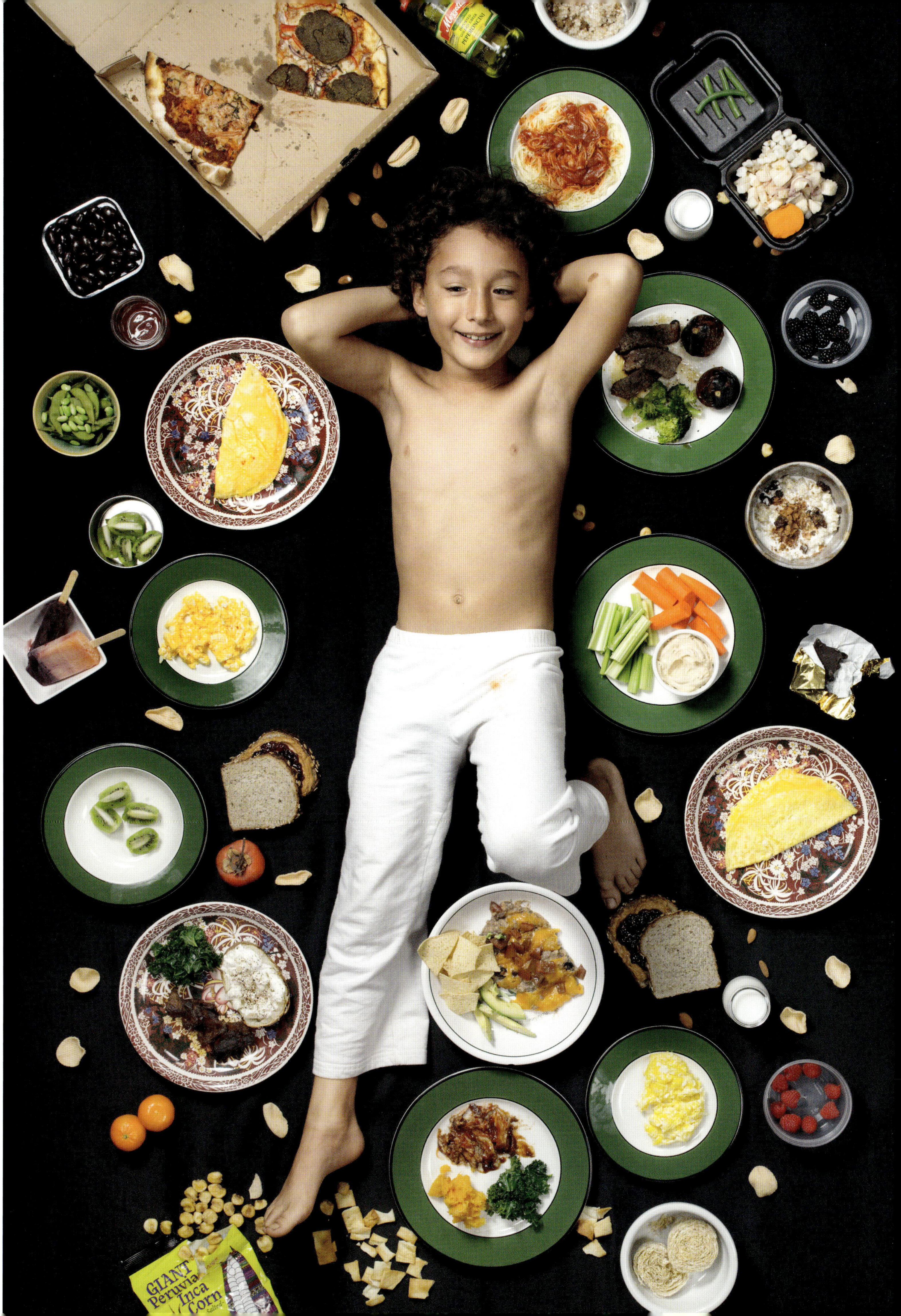
GIANT
Peruvia
Inca
Corn

Agata Grasso, 9

Catania, Sicily, Italy.
Photographed August 23, 2017.

Agata lives in an apartment in Catania with her father, a mason, her mother, a housewife, and her 6-year-old sister. In Agata's house, the food is always made by her mother, except for Saturday nights when they order a pizza or eat out. Agata isn't fond of fish, but loves mashed potatoes and sweet foods like muffins and little chocolate lava cakes, which she's learned to make herself. Her earliest memory of food is the spaghetti with squid ink her mom made—and how her face and hands were soiled with the oily black sauce. Agata loves to sing, collects figurines, and cherishes her dog Charly. She likes romantic stories, like her grandparents' love story: her grandmother worked in a shop. One day, her grandfather entered and was struck by her beauty. To see her again, he came every day to the store to buy something. This went on for weeks. Before becoming poor, her grandfather found courage and told her he was in love with her and they were engaged. If she had enough money, Agata would buy a villa for her family.

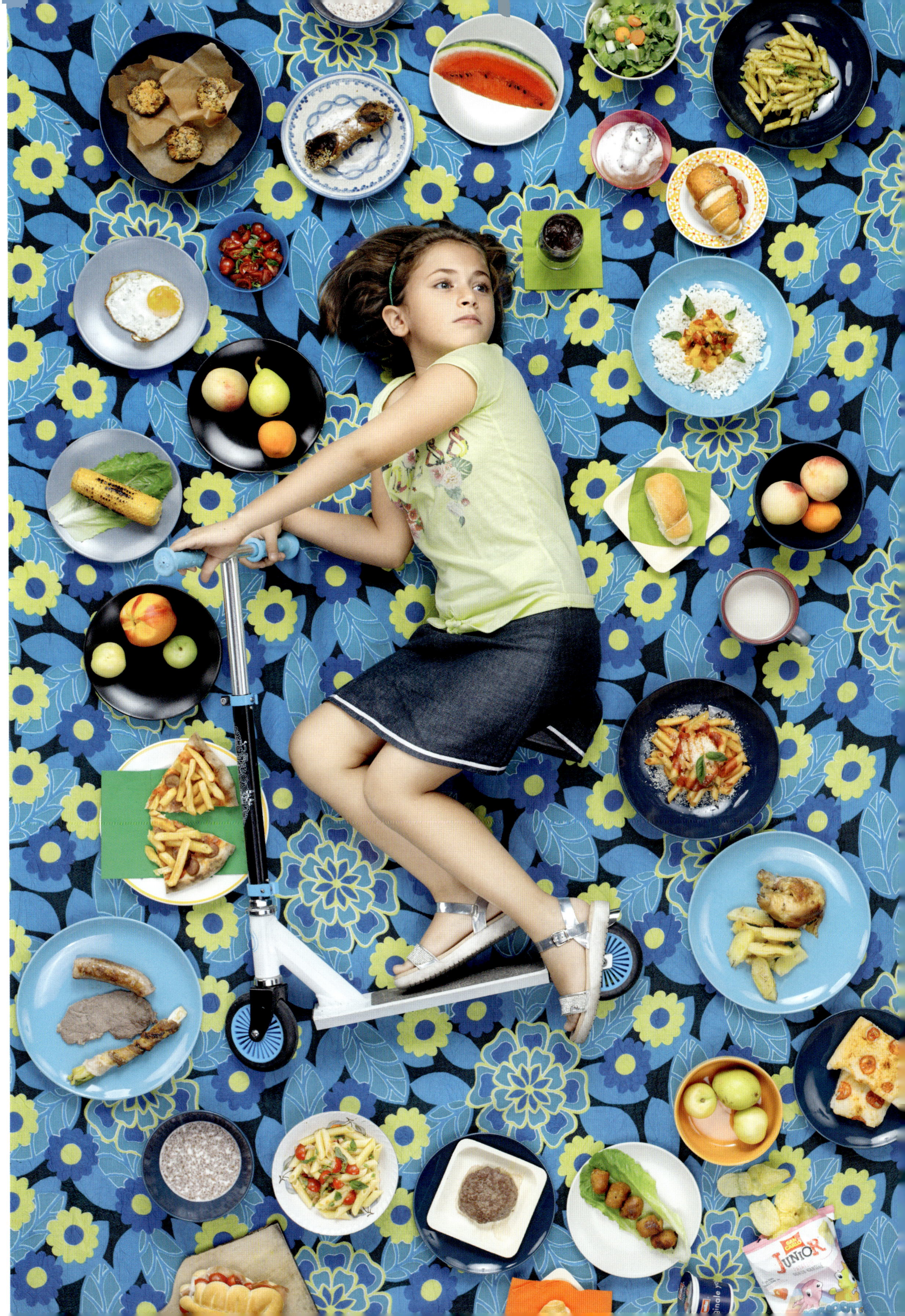
JUNIOR

Prince Miller, 13

Los Angeles, CA, USA.
Photographed March 19, 2016.

When he was 12, Prince and his family left St. James Montego Bay for the US. His parents decided life in Jamaica was too dangerous after Prince's cousin was gunned down at the little neighborhood market the family owned. Prince misses the green open space of his family farm and the animals they raised: goats, chickens, geese, rabbits, pigs, and cows. Two rivers irrigated the property where they grew and harvested corn, yams, coconuts, oranges, apples, pears, ackee, and breadfruit. Prince misses his dad, too, who's stuck in Montego Bay driving a cab. Prince's diet isn't as healthy as it was in Jamaica, but he'll try just about anything. His favorite dishes are sushi, fried chicken, and Chinese barbeque which he gets on special occasions. On Fridays, Prince helps prepare the family dinner, usually sausage, rice, broccoli, and salad. Prince's cousins say he ought to be a therapist because he's a good listener, but his sights are set on playing pro football. He's been scouted by colleges already and has run 100 meters in 11.49 seconds. When he goes to sleep at night, Prince mostly prays to Jesus that crime and cheating will be less throughout the world and that his dad will get his papers and come to America. He wishes, too, that he'll be able to buy his mother another farm someday.

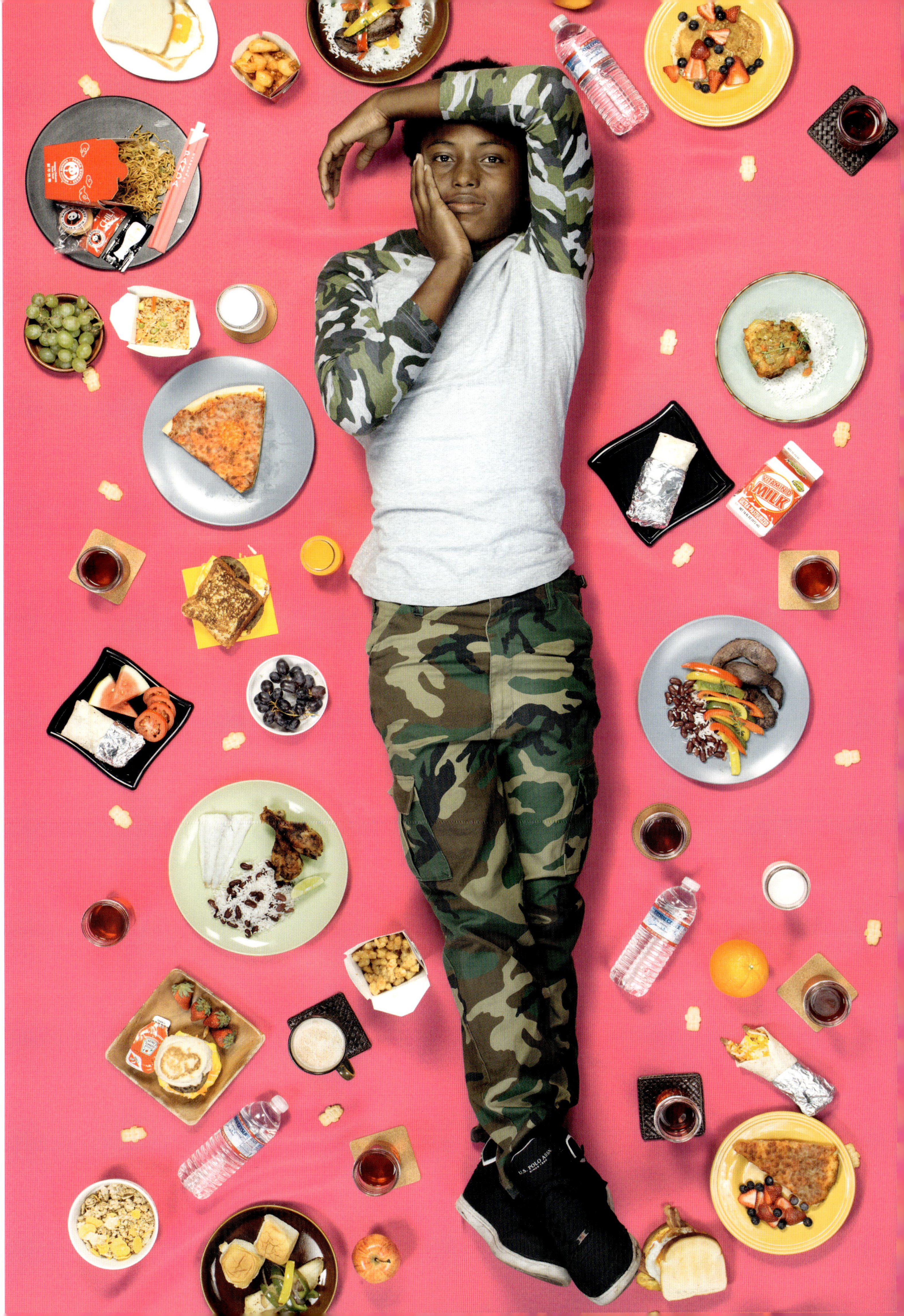
MILK

Leona "Nona" Del Grosso Sands, 6

Glendale, CA, USA.
Photographed January 30, 2016.

Nona lives with her mother and Cleo, her beloved cat, in an apartment in Glendale, California. She can make oatmeal and pancakes and once when her mother was very sick, she fed her. Nona grew a gigantic tomato plant that began to take over everything and is now as big as a tree. Her mother makes her eat vegetables, especially broccoli. Her diet has as many colors as the rainbow, though Nona also has not just a sweet tooth, but many "sugar teeth." Nona's role models are her mother, her teachers, and Joan Jett. When she goes to sleep at night, Nona sometimes imagines her Nana is an angel watching over her.

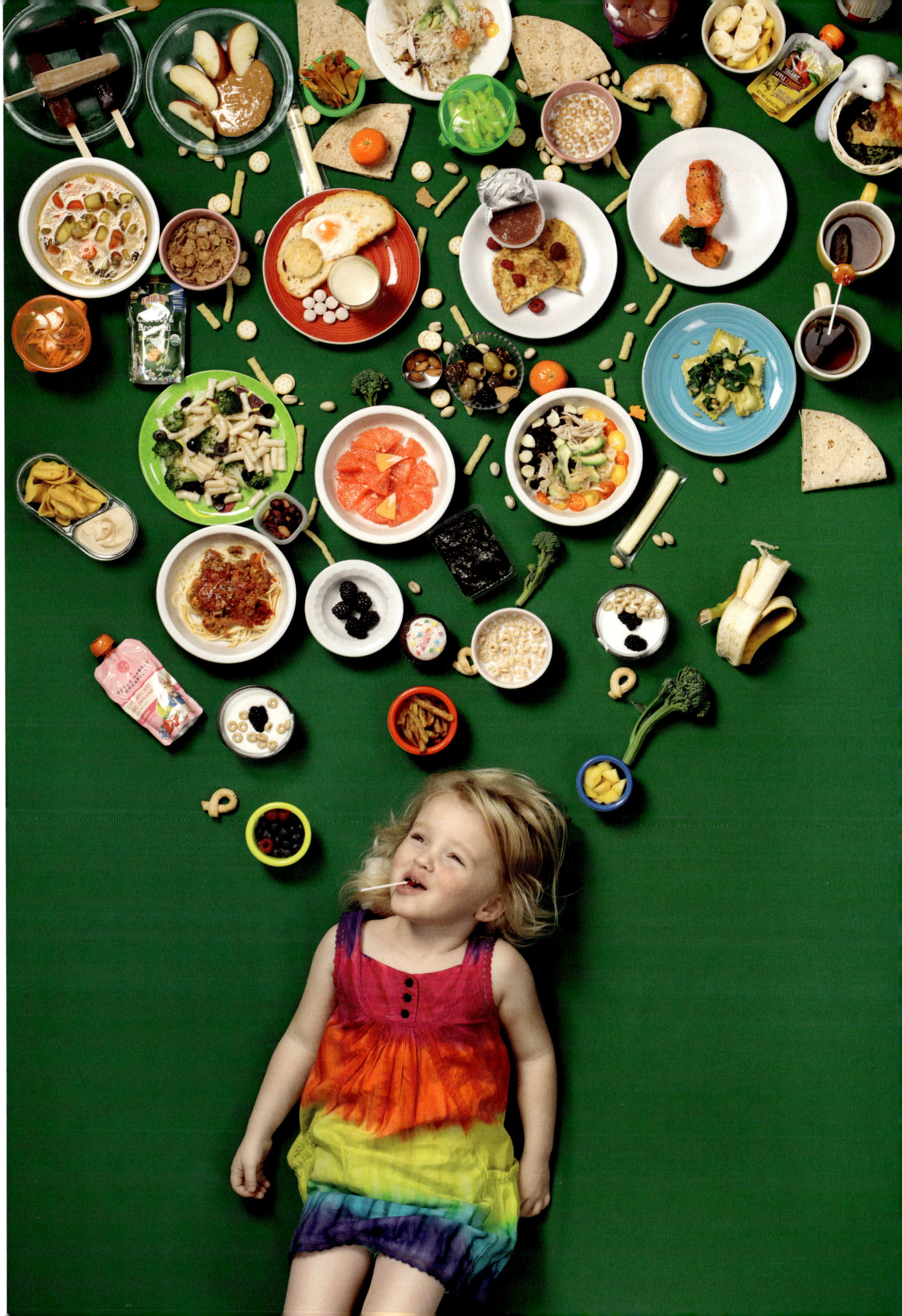

Joshua Poulain, 12

La Colle-sur-Loup, France.
Photographed August 18, 2017 in Nice.

Josh lives with his parents and younger brother in La Colle-sur-Loup, a resort town ten minutes outside Nice. From his bedroom window, Josh can see the forest and hills of Col de Vence and the family garden where they grow tomatoes, peppers, zucchini, and onions. Josh's pop is a locksmith and his mom is an accountant. He eats four times a day and his favorite dish is his mother's lasagna. The only foods he dislikes are fish and bananas. There are two rules for mealtimes: no phones and you can't leave the table till you've cleaned your plate. Josh can cook pasta but prefers baking cakes with his mom. When he's on holiday, he eats plenty of junk food. Josh's favorite smell is his grandmother's perfume and the only thing missing in his life is his dead cat. Josh wishes he could play basketball like Steph Curry or Tony Parker. If he had enough money he'd buy a motorcycle. He'd like to keep his blankie forever and someday be a Lego designer. One thing characterizes Josh's family: no one leaves home without saying "I love you."

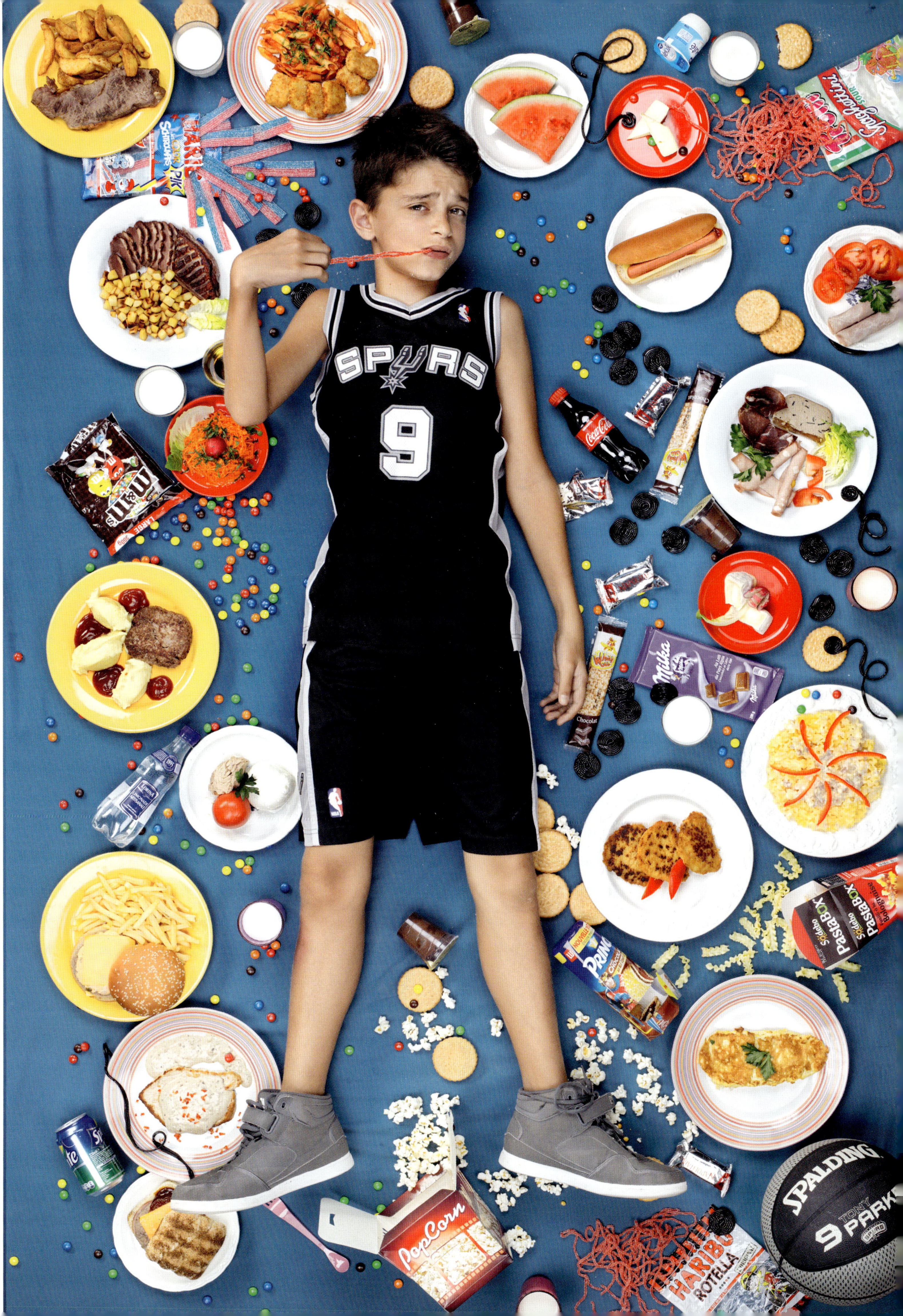
SPURS
9
Milka
PopCorn
HARIBO
ROTELLA
SPALDING
PastaBOX

Razan Habib, 11

Ajman, UAE.
Photographed August 12, 2018 in Dubai.

Razan lives in a quiet neighborhood on the outskirts of Dubai with her mother. There is only desert around them. Villas, cars, dogs, cats, and desert sand. Razan's mom works long hours as an events coordinator, and as a single mom, doesn't have time to cook most days, so most often, they eat out. Razan thinks she has a healthy diet, but her mom disagrees: "I'm putting everything in front of her, but she's not eating. She's not interested in vegetables. She likes this junk food that is full of bread, carbohydrates. If I force her to eat the vegetables, she will not eat. Whatever will come with force will not remain. I wish her mind will be more open." Razan's favorite food is a Whopper with plenty of pickles. Sometimes Razan is naughty and teases her classmates. She idolizes Christian Ronaldo. She loves jewelry, makeup, and her mobile. Most nights, she falls asleep watching YouTube videos.

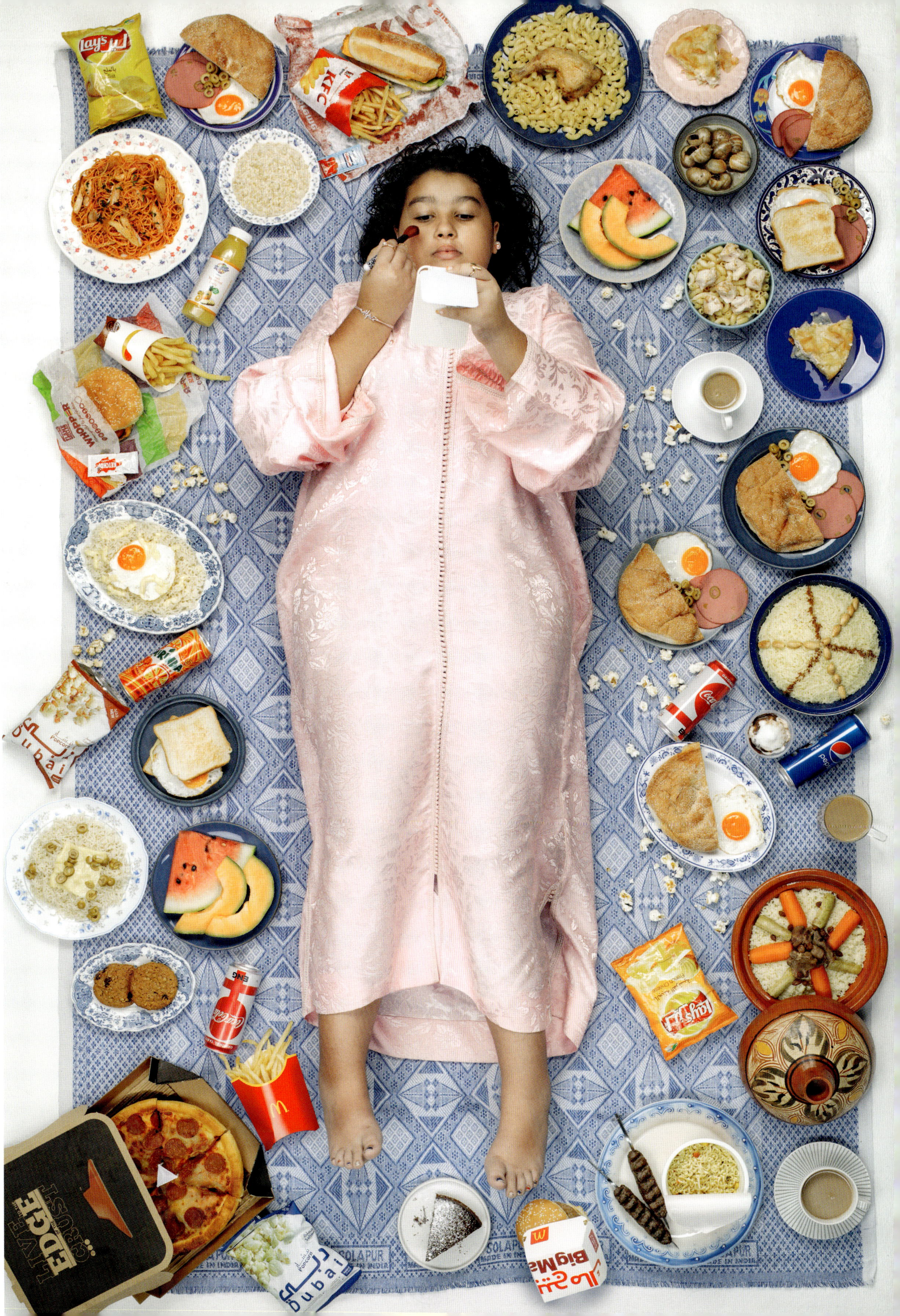
Lay's
KFC
WHOPPER
Coca-Cola
Pepsi
LIVE EDGE CRUST
Big Mac
SOLAPUR
MADE IN INDIA

Shraman Gaware, 12

Mumbai, India.
Photographed March 12, 2017.

Shraman, an only child, lives with his mom, a housewife, and dad, a municipal officer, in a middle-class Mumbai high-rise surrounded by slums. Shraman loves spicy barbe-que chicken, burgers, pizza, poha (a puffed rice snack), timok (a rice flour pancake served with lentil curry), and street food from the Chinese stalls in his neighborhood. At home, Shraman makes pasta and tea for himself. He has never grown his own food, though once, while visiting his uncle in Nasik, a village about 200 kms north of Mumbai, he harvested corn. He was impressed by the towering plants and helped his uncle pluck, shuck, and eat the corn. Shraman collects copies of *Tinkle* a kid's magazine filled with jokes and puzzles and watches soccer on his smart phone. Shraman has a talent for singing, cracking jokes, and making ridiculous faces. He would like to be a stand-up comedian or actor. If he had extra money he would save it for a rainy day.

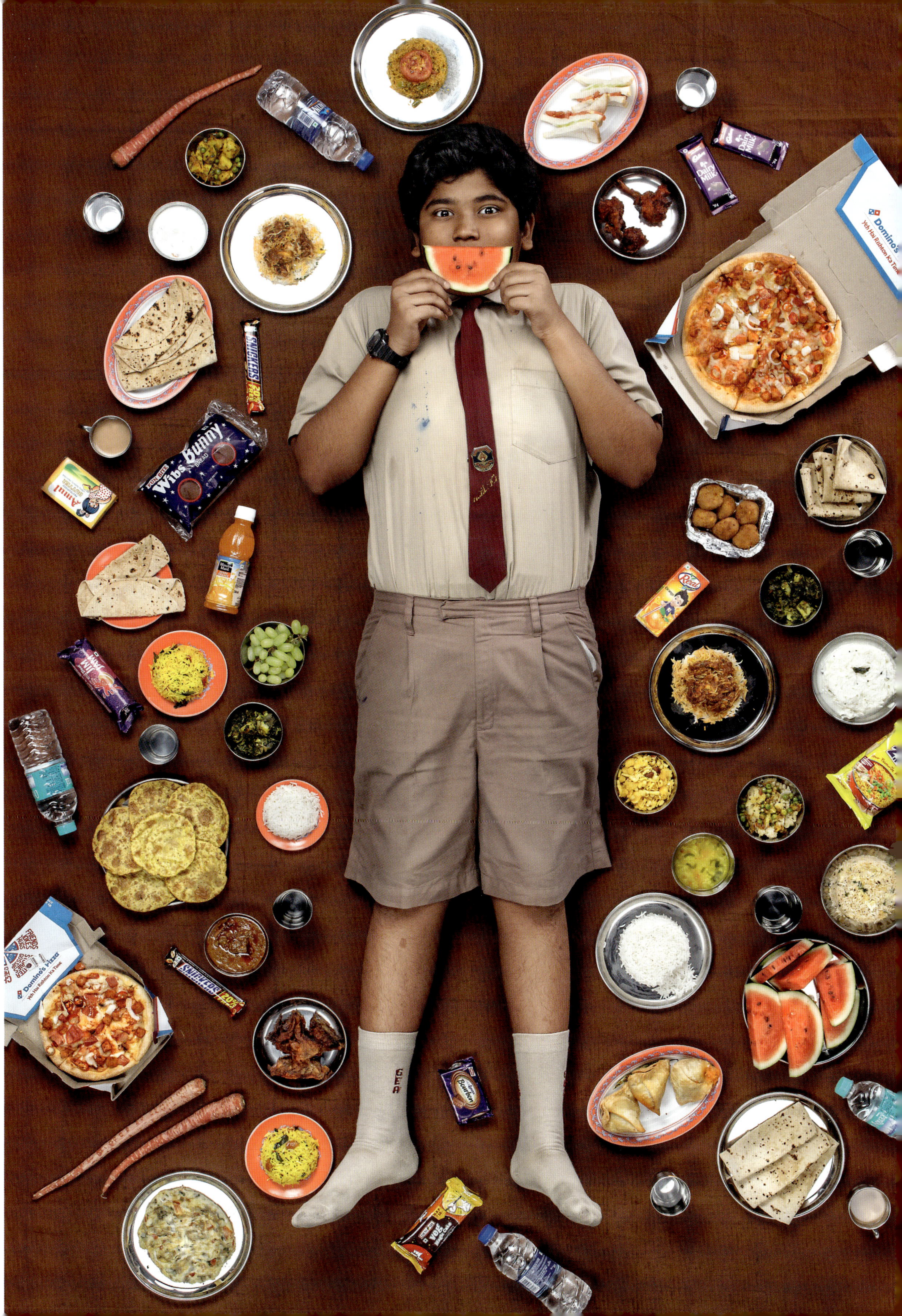
Domino's
Yeh Hai Rishton Ka Time
Dairy Milk
Wibs Bunny
Amul
Snickers
Real
Domino's Pizza
Bourbon

Kaira Mbodji, 7

Dakar, Senegal.
Photographed August 30, 2017.

Kaira lives with her mum and dad, mammy, cousins, and aunties in Amitié 3, a quiet, middle-class neighborhood in western Dakar a few blocks from the Atlantic Ocean where, on a Sunday, you might find shepherds bathing and manicuring their sheep. Rams and sheep are everywhere in Dakar, kept inside homes as companion animals. In Kaira's home, mum and aunties do the cooking and only occasionally does the family eat out. Kaira's favorite food is pasta and she's learning to cook; pancakes are her specialty. In her backyard, the family has a small garden with a lemon tree and beans growing on vines. Kaira goes to Poucinet, a cheerful yellow private school with French and Senegalese flags flying in front. Kaira loves skateboarding and making up dance moves to hip-hop or mbalax (which means rhythm in Wolof, the Senegalese language). Kaira collects shoes and the pink and black Adidas she's wearing in the photo are her favorite pair.

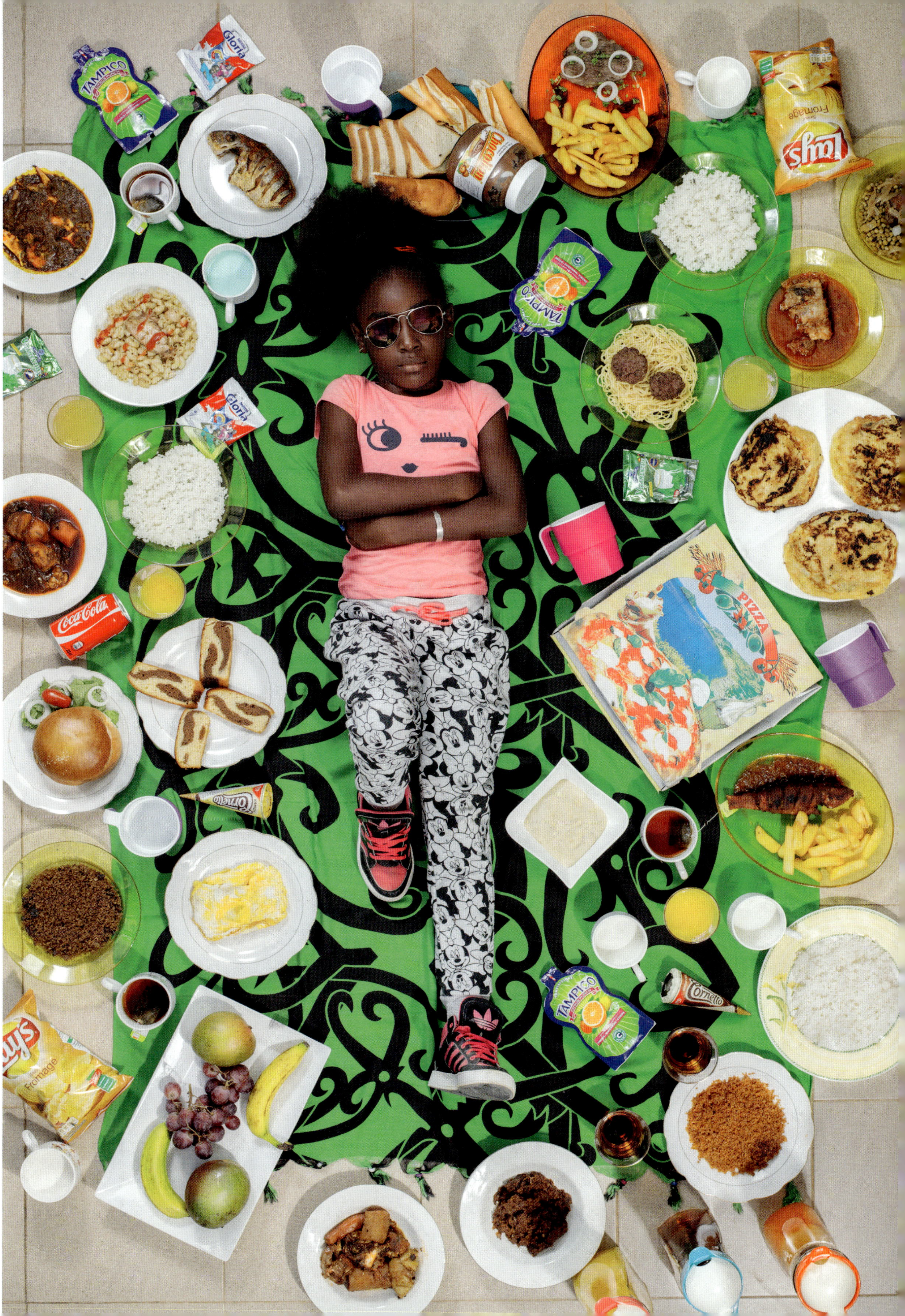
TAMPICO
Gloria
Lay's
Fromage
Coca-Cola
PIZZA
Cornetto

Rayirth Gupta, 10

Mumbai, India.
Photographed March 12, 2017.

Rayirth was born in the US, but after his parents separated, his mom brought him to Mumbai to raise him with the help of her parents. Quiet and soft spoken, Rayirth eats large quantities of nuts, legumes, fruits, and vegetables and loves all his granny's home-cooked meals. His earliest food memory is of eating khichadi, a typical Indian dish made with rice and lentils and served with yogurt. The family seldom eats out. Once in a while, Rayirth craves a pizza, but this is a rare treat; mostly, junk food is off-limits. Rayirth was astonished by the quantity of food he consumes in a week and proud that his diet is healthier than most of his friends. Rayirth plays cricket, badminton, and classical guitar; takes life-drawing classes; and collects postage stamps. He loves their colors and designs, especially the ones from distant places. If Rayirth had enough money, he'd travel throughout India and abroad, collecting stamps from each place he visits. Before sleep, Rayirth watches animal videos on his mobile with his mom for 15 minutes. When the lights are turned out, he prays for her to be healthy and happy and hopes he will make her proud. He will follow in his mother's footsteps because he admires her and what she has achieved.

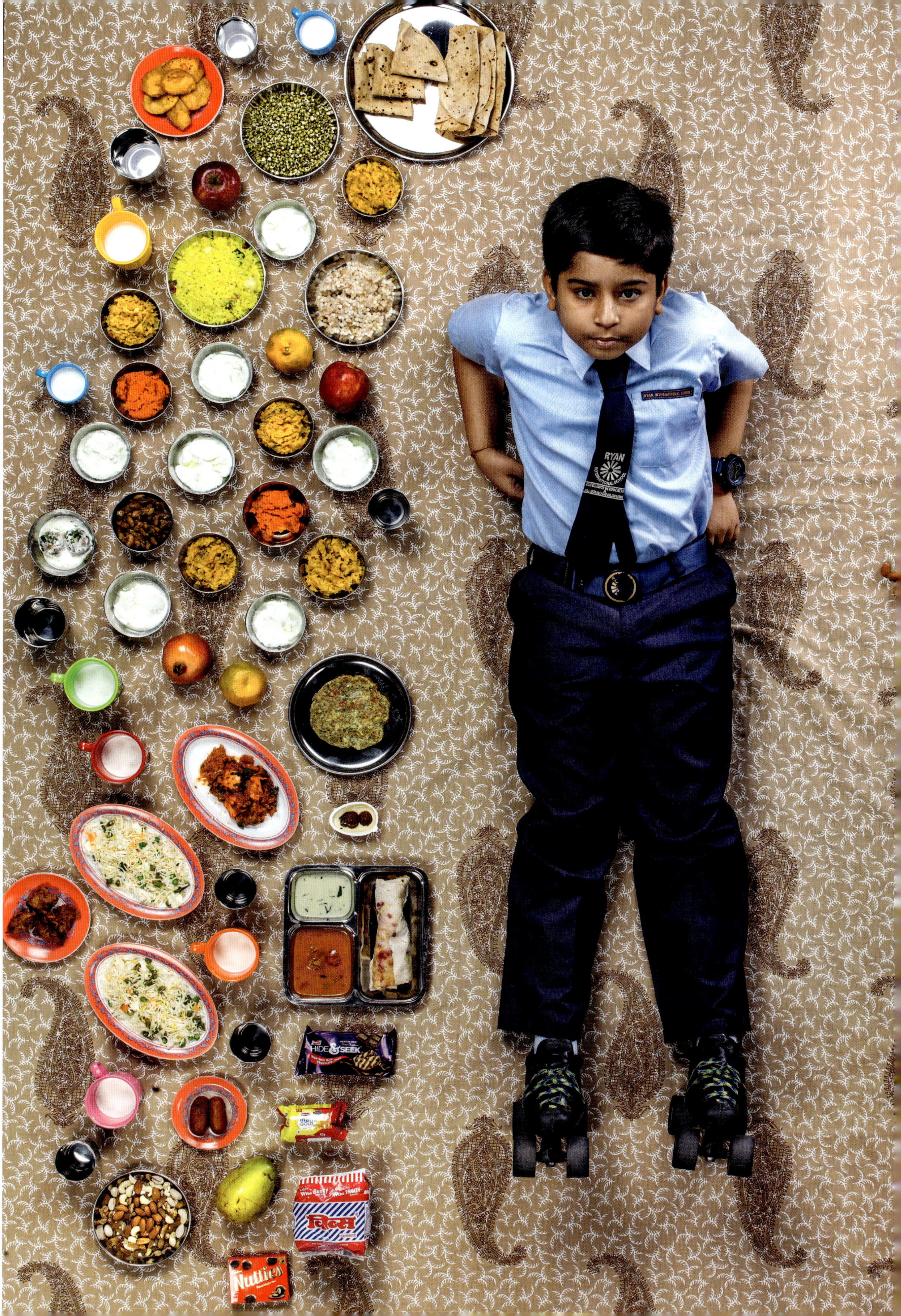
HIDE & SEEK
Nutties
RYAN

Siti Khaliesah Nataliea Muhamad Khairizal, 9

Kuala Lumpur, Malaysia.
Photographed March 26, 2017.

Siti lives in a suburb of Kuala Lumpur with her father, a car salesman, her mother, a housewife, and her four siblings. Mum does all the cooking and sets the rules for the table: recite the du'a, no water before meals, and no chatting during meals, though it's very seldom that the whole family sits down to dinner together because everyone's so busy. Siti's favorite dish is spaghetti carbonara and she's crazy about the scent of fried instant noodles. She goes to a Chinese school where she learns Mandarin, plays the melodian, and practices taekwando. When she falls asleep at night, Siti wishes her dad would put some money under her pillow. She collects coins of all kinds and foreign currencies. Once she saves enough money, Siti's going to buy an iPad.

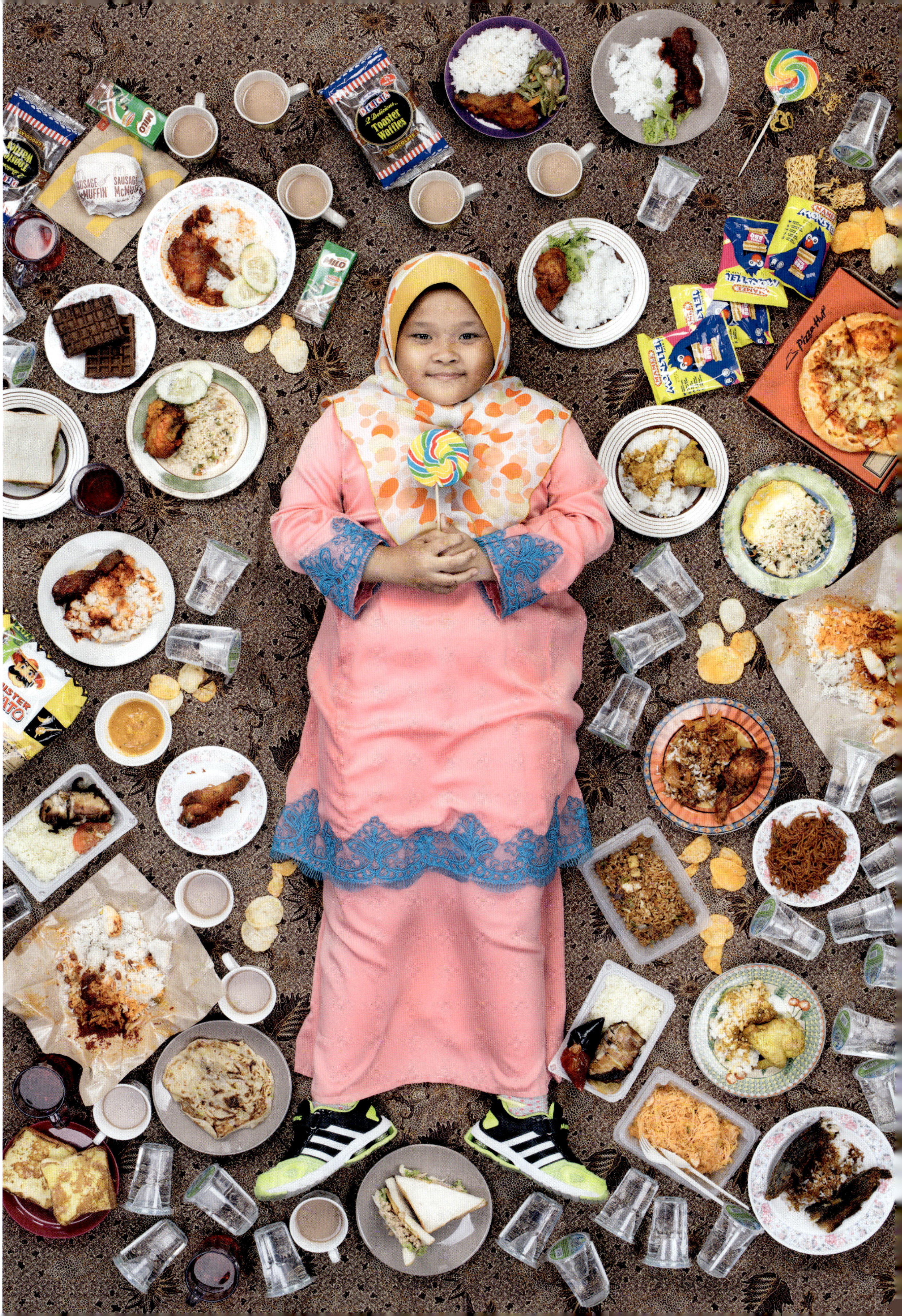
Toaster Waffles
MILO
Pizza Hut

Ana Rodriguez, 16

Los Angeles, CA, USA.
Photographed March 21, 2016.

At the time of the photo shoot, Ana lived with her grandparents in Westlake, a Central-American neighborhood near downtown Los Angeles. One hundred thousand people are crammed into three square miles and the dirty, neglected streets have long been gang turf, graffiti scrawl everywhere.

Ana's earliest memories of food are the family potlucks, the house filled with cousins, aunts, uncles, and grandparents, everyone bringing a dish: pupusas, tamales, and tres leches cake. Ana isn't a picky eater. She loves spicy Thai noodles, scallop rolls, and tuna sushi. After posing with her food, Ana saw what was missing in her diet: fresh greens. The problem is, "You won't see a Whole Foods where I live. You can find plenty of liquor stores, but it's hard to find fresh fruits and vegetables, especially organic!"

Ana is active in her community, volunteering with non-profit organizations and feeding the homeless. For her, it's a way of restoring humanity to the community and debunking stereotypes. Her role model has always been her grandmother, who taught her empathy and resilience and sacrificed so much. Even now, she scrapes by on retirement but still helps Ana with school costs. Now a sophmore at UC Berkeley, Ana majors in social welfare and gender studies. She plans to be a public defender, working with disadvantaged minorities. When she goes to sleep at night, Ana thinks about her future and how she can support her siblings in their academics. She knows that college is a way out of poverty, yet it isn't something talked about in her family.

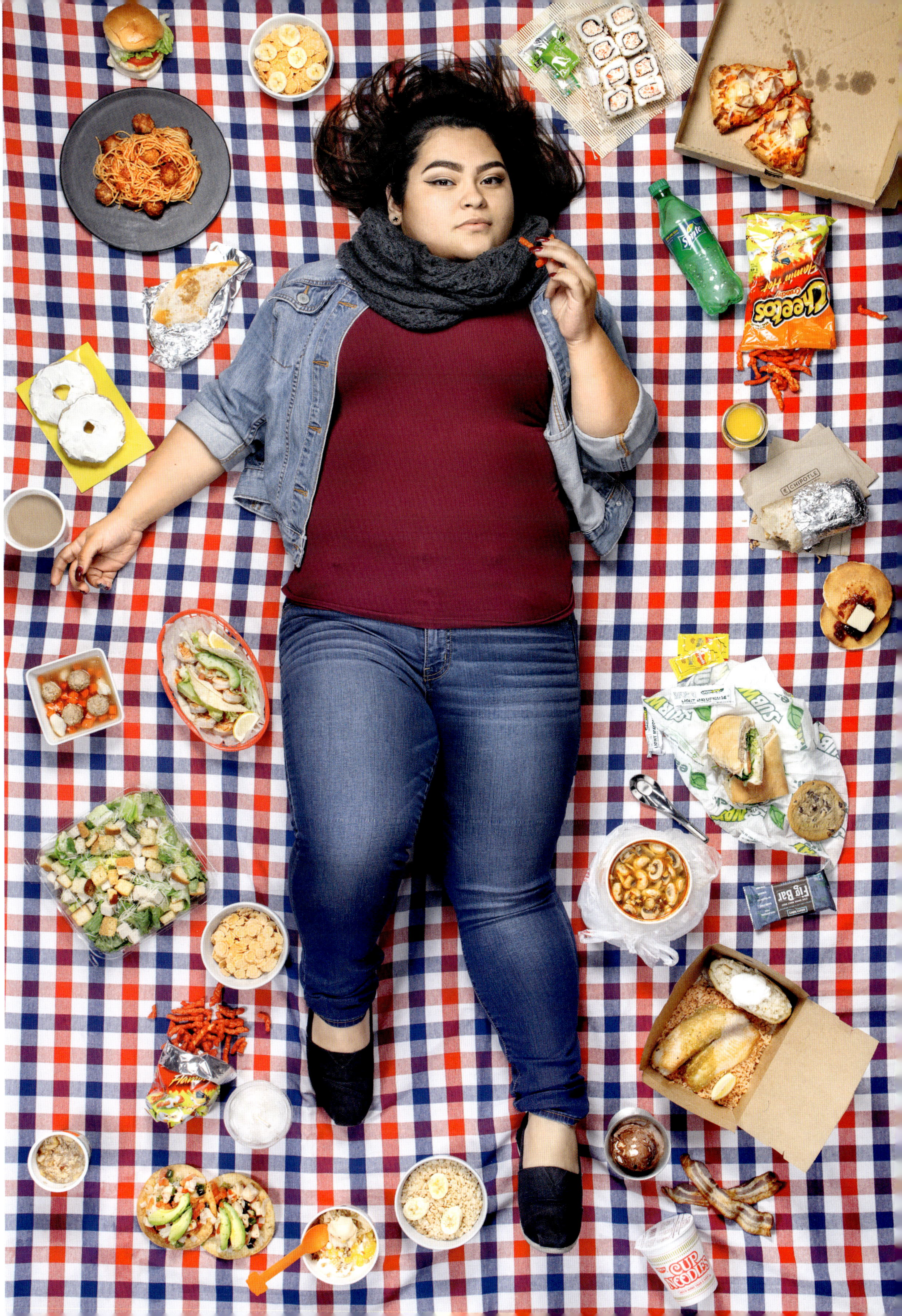
Sprite
Cheetos
CHIPOTLE
SUBWAY
Fig Bar
CUP NOODLES

Lily Tyteca, 8

Nice, France.
Photographed August 18, 2017.

Lily, an only child, lives part time with her mom, a makeup artist, and dad, a network technician. From her dad's apartment, she looks out onto a flower shop and a funeral parlor. From her mom's place, her view is of a driving school and car repair shop. She goes to St. Barthelemy's and excels in English and fitness. All of Lily's meals are home-cooked, never store bought. Her earliest memory of food is the taste of spinach. Since then, Lily has grown and harvested tomatoes, green beans, strawberries, raspberries, asparagus, thyme, lettuce, and zucchini. But her favorite food is a hamburger. Lily loves to go rock climbing with her dad. She comes from a long line of tough men: her grandfather Charlie was a warrior in Algeria and her great-grandfather was in the big war. They're both still alive. When she's older, Lily will either work to protect the rights of animals or be a gym teacher. If she were wealthy, she would buy a beautiful house and donate the rest to children's charities. Lily falls asleep to the music of Ariana Grande and collects snow globes from around the world. She wishes that her parents would never cry.

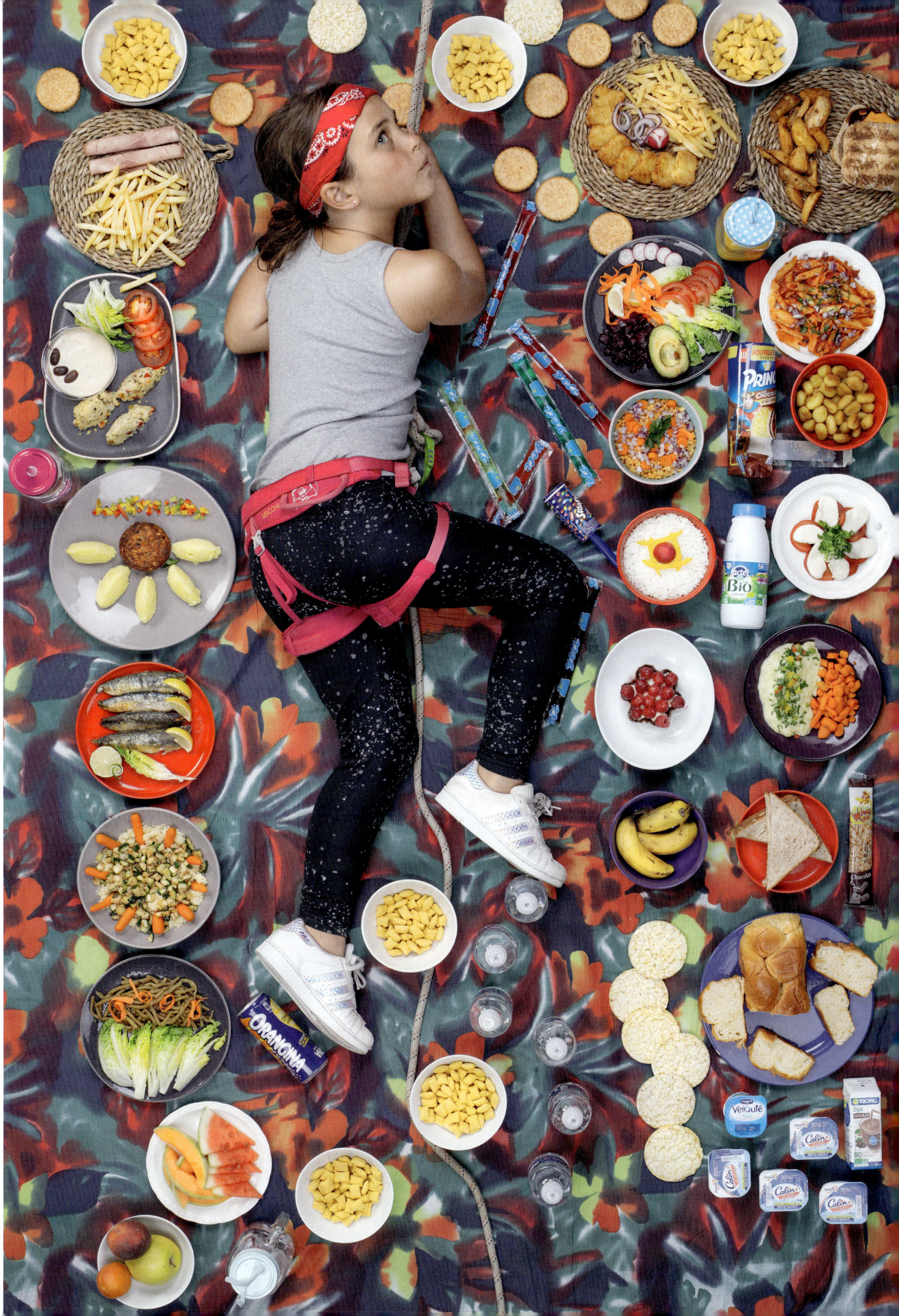
ORANGINA
Bio
Velouté
BJORG

John Hintze, 7

Hamburg, Germany.
Photographed August 11, 2017.

John lives with his parents in a large apartment with a garden in a quiet suburb of Hamburg with more trees than cars. John describes himself as an omnivore. He's fond of eating breakfast in bed. His parents bring him a tray of muesli and toast every morning before school. John loves his grandma's roast, Chinese curry with cashew nuts, and Orange Fanta, though he's only allowed to drink Fanta on weekends. During the week there is only water. He used to like mushrooms, but not anymore. Once, with his friend Henry, he made a fruit plate with a sushi knife. "I have not yet harvested something to eat, but I could do that. First we'd have to plant something." John collects minerals like purple azurite, is learning Thai kickboxing, sailing, and is an accomplished swimmer. He would like to be an underwater archeologist. His dad has already found and brought back great things from the sea. Once, when he and his dad were snorkeling, a curious octopus approached them—which was both scary and fantastic. When he falls asleep at night, John paints a mental picture of what will happen tomorrow. He hopes his parents will never die.

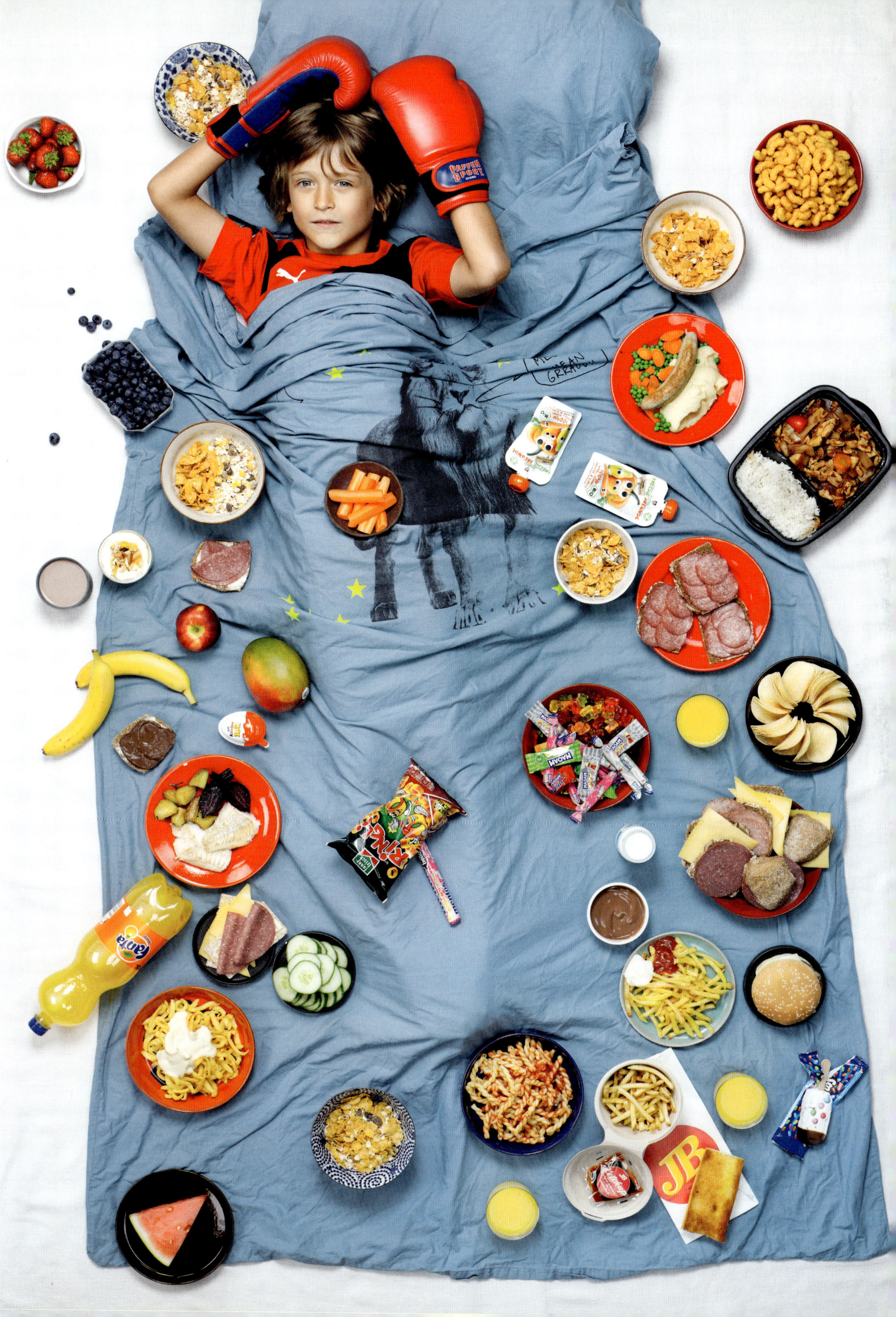
Fanta
JB

Tharkish Sri Ganesh and Mierra Sri Varrsha, 10 and 8

Bukit Jalil, Malaysia.
Photographed March 26, 2017.

Tharkish and Mierra's roots in Malaysia begin with their great-grandfather who migrated from South India to build a better future, but only found work as a rubber tapper before being conscripted by the Japanese to build the "Death Railway" from Thailand to Myanmar in 1943. Tharkish and Mierra live with their mom and dad in a public housing project in Bukit Jalil, a suburb of Kuala Lumpur. Their apartment block is full of friends and noisy in a good way. Their dad works as a gaffer in film production and their mom is a homemaker and does most of the cooking, though on weekends they eat KFC, Pizza Hut, or get Chinese takeout. Mierra dislikes the pungent smell of meat and traces of blood. She prefers candies and chocolates. Her earliest memory of food is rice porridge, her comfort food whenever she falls sick. Tharkish's favorite food is puttu, steamed ground rice layered with coconut and topped with bananas and palm sugar. Tharkish doesn't like onions because they taste weird and leave a funny smell in his mouth. His first taste was urad dal porridge, an Indian baby food made with dal, rice, coconut, cardamon, and jaggery (concentrated date palm sap). Mierra says her diet is healthy because her mom avoids foods with preservatives, additives, and MSG, though after her Daily Bread portrait, she still thinks she could eat less processed food. Mierra loves to read and play badminton and Snakes and Ladders while her brother is into chess, carom, and surfing the internet. Mierra strives to be the top student in her class and wants to be a doctor while Tharkish will be happy with a top three finish after examinations and pictures himself as an IT engineer.

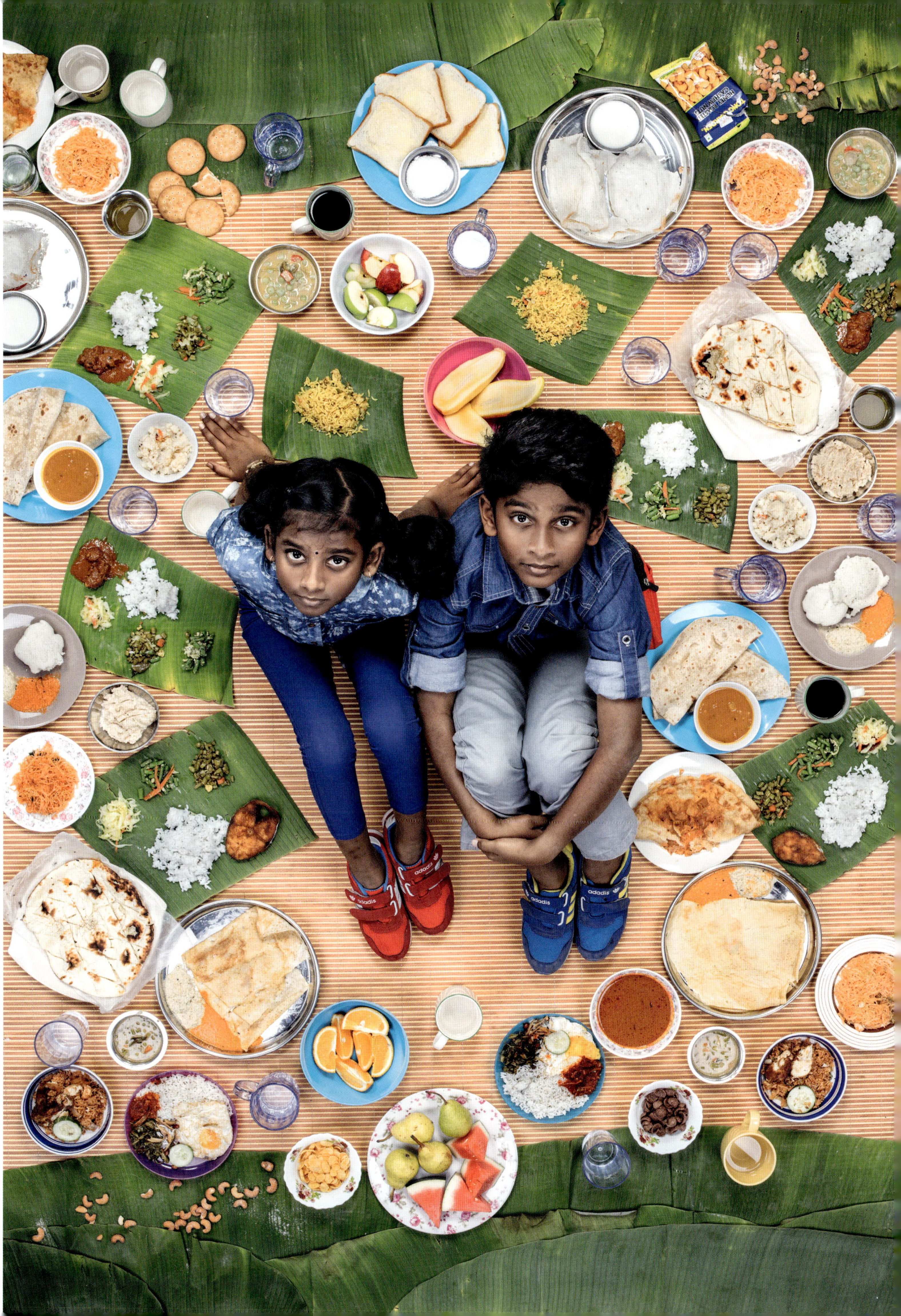

Acknowledgements

Daily Bread would not have been possible without the team at powerHouse Books: Daniel Power, founder, Craig Cohen, executive publisher, and designer Kris Pulochowicz.

I'm grateful for the recognition and support I've received from the many magazines and newspapers around the world that have published *Daily Bread*. I'm particularly appreciative of support from *Time* magazine and Deputy Director of Photography Paul Moakley who sponsored my Dakar shoot and *Geo* Germany and Photo Editor Peter Unterthurner who sponsored my Hamburg shoot.

My gratitude goes out to the producers in each of the countries I visited, whose assistance in networking with families and organizing the photo shoots was essential: Namrata Paralker in Mumbai, Venkatesh Somasundaram in Kuala Lumpur, Hanne Evans in Nice, Maurizio Licciardello in Catania, Meissa Seck in Dakar, Wild Media in Dubai, and Pablo Roy and Marcelo Barki in Brazil. I owe a debt of gratitude to Anna Penido and Denise Barbosa Silva for sharing their knowledge of indigenous Brazilian culture and native foods, and connecting me with families living in remote regions of the country.

A heartfelt thanks to the cooks and food stylists who worked long and hard to recreate each of the children's menus. Alyssa Noui, Elena Vega, Iman Kawa, and Angie Su in Los Angeles; Volker Hobl and Julia Luck in

Hamburg; Cuisine Riviera and Samyra Fakhoury in Nice; Raffaella Esposito in Catania; Soukheyna Sagna in Dakar; Mary-Kei Macfarlane in Dubai; and Tainá Förthmann and Ana Paula Boquadi in São Paolo.

My gratitude also goes out to the generous and talented Gretchen Hilmers/G-Tou who prepared all my images for publication and to Dana Kozeff whose expertise and resourcefulness in many roles made my Los Angeles shoots a success.

I'm grateful also to my Kickstarter supporters who helped make it possible to broaden the scope of the project to India and Malayasia.

I'm honored to have received the 2018 Food Sustainability Media Award, organized by Thomson Reuters Foundation and Barilla Center for Food and Nutrition Foundation.

A huge thank you to all the children and parents of *Daily Bread*, who enlarged my world and made the project a success.

And the hugest thank you of all to my toughest critic and biggest supporter, my wife Dani Palomino.

Daily Bread:
What Kids Eat Around the World

Published in the United States by powerHouse Books, a division of powerHouse Cultural Entertainment, Inc.
32 Adams Street, Brooklyn, NY 11201-1021
e-mail: info@powerHouseBooks.com
website: www.powerHouseBooks.com

First edition, 2019

Library of Congress Control Number: 2018968128

ISBN 978-1-57687-911-5

Designed by Krzysztof Poluchowicz

Printed by Pimlico Book International

10 9 8 7 6 5 4 3 2

Printed and bound in China